# Through My Eyes

## A Mother's Guide from Baby

*Through My Eyes. A Mother's Guide from Baby* by Marie Rosier
Photography by Julieanne Perara
Published by Australian eBook Publisher
www.AustralianEbookPublisher.com.au


1st Edition 2016, pbk.
ISBN: 978-1-925516-32-6
Designer: Sharnai James-McGovern, Australian eBook Publisher

**National Library of Australia Cataloguing-in-Publication Entry:**

| | |
|---|---|
| Creator: | Rosier, Marie, author. |
| Title: | Through my eyes : a mother's guide from baby / Marie Rosier ; photographer: Julieanne Perara. |
| ISBN: | 9781925516326 (paperback)<br>9781925516302 (ebook : epub)<br>9781925516319 (ebook : mobi) |
| Subjects: | Infants--Care.<br>Child rearing.<br>Parenting.<br>Parent and child. |
| Other Creators/ Contributors: | Perara, Julieanne, photographer. |
| Dewey Number: | 649.122 |

Also available as an ebook from major ebook vendors.

**Find the author at rosieroutlook.com.au**

# Through My Eyes

## A Mother's Guide from Baby

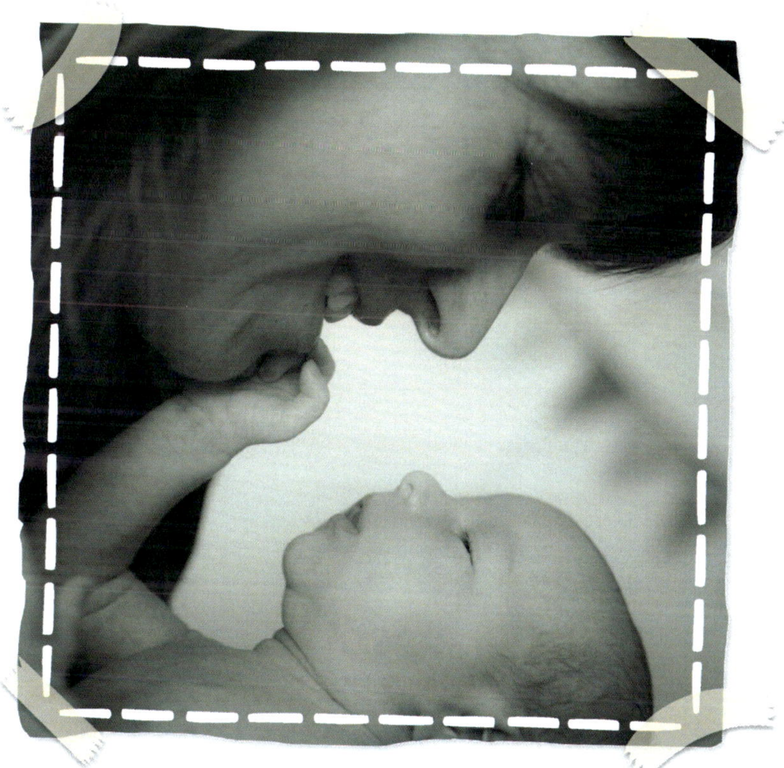

Written by Marie Rosier

Photography by Julieanne Perara

'There is only one task and that is to increase the store of love within us.'

—Tolstoy

# Dedication

This book is dedicated to all mothers of the world, especially the women of the Kopanang project in South Africa. Just over 80 women and their dependents, numbering nearly 600, find hope there. They survive amidst relentless struggles of domestic violence, rape, HIV/AIDS and extreme poverty.

When mothering gets challenging for those of us in calmer places, let them be our inspiration. After all, we are all sisters united in motherhood and raising our children in the best way we can.

(See page 91 for more about Kopanang)

## About Marie Rosier

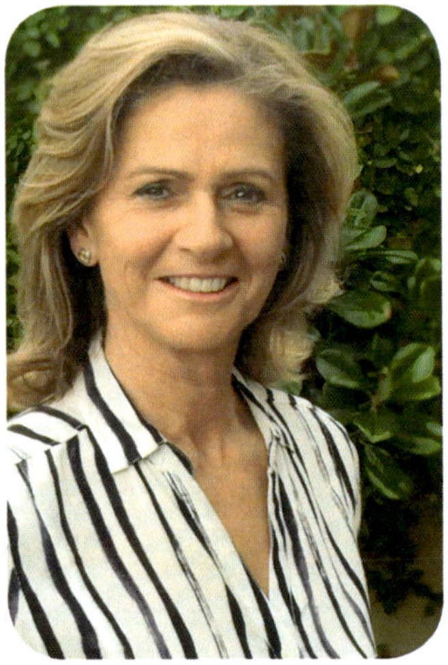

Marie Rosier is a Coach, Counsellor, Psychotherapist and Educator. In private practice in Melbourne, Australia and through seminars she enables people to develop their capacity to manage life's challenges more effectively and live more joyfully. She is passionate about her work with parents, especially mothers—to raise happy and resilient children.

rosieroutlook.com.au

## About Julieanne Perara

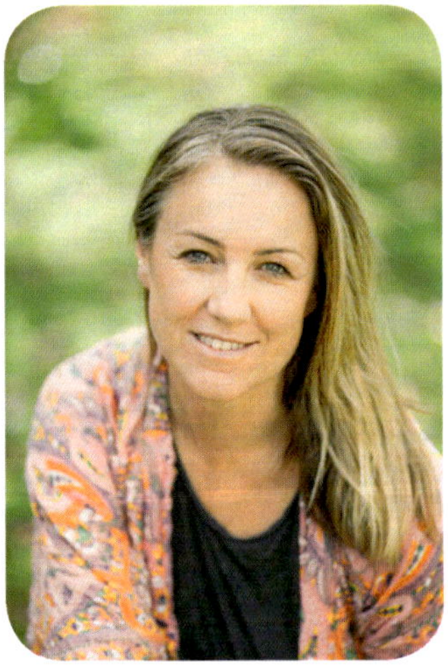

Julieanne Perara is a wonderfully gifted photographer; a romantic at heart with a love for capturing beautiful moments that result in images that reveal the depths of human beauty and vulnerability.

julieanneperaraphotography.com.au

# Foreword

We know so much, and yet so little, about the intimate attachment between mothers and babies. One certainty is the importance of this bond throughout life. In this delightful book, Marie Rosier draws on developmental psychology, her work as a psychotherapist and her own experience, in imagining the world of the newborn child. Marie invites you to join her in her exploration of the world of mothers and their babies.

—Dr Coral Brown FAPS Assistant Director
The Cairnmillar Institute

# Preface

The aim of this book is to help mothers develop awareness, understanding and an appreciation of the hugely beneficial role they can play in promoting their babies' healthy development.

Although written for new mothers, it will benefit anyone caring for a baby, such as partners and grandparents.

Following 25 years working with people of all ages in education, business, psychotherapy and counselling, I have come to know and see the huge impact that our early years, particularly those with our mother, have on the person we become; how we are to enjoy life and manage what it throws at us.

Within you'll find power-packed little nuggets of information and some strategies to try. The content arises from my client work, research and bringing up my own children, which I joke have provided me with an informal laboratory. Yet it was my top signature strength, 'to love and be loved' that was the ultimate guide that led to the words that make my heart sing... and I hope yours will too.

For this reason and as a gift to my five adult children who are embarking on their own parenting journeys, I present to you this book of gems. You'll find important material from sources reaching far and wide. This includes facts from the cutting-edge field of neuroscience and its breakthrough discoveries around brain plasticity—our brains' ability to develop and change after influence from deep connection with those closest to us, particularly the bond between mother, baby and the environment.

To make for an easy and enjoyable read, this book avoids in-depth information or scientific jurgon. It does not aim in providing answers for babies or mothers who are experiencing extreme challenges. That is best referred to professionals on a more personal level. No, "this is the magic book" as it was described by one of our gorgeous mothers photographed. This book seeks to warm and open your heart to promote the development of a beautiful bond between you and your baby.

A living project morphed beyond its original scope, this book has already connected people in ways that I could not have envisaged at the start. Thank you to all who helped bring it to fruition and those in my life that simply left a bit of their sparkle on me.

Heartfelt thanks to my family: Norman, Christina, Lauren, Gavan, Samantha and Jacqueline, for enriching my life and supporting me in my work. Thankyou to all the mothers, babies, fathers, brothers and sisters who appear in this book and were so beautifully photographed by the talented, Julieanne Perara. Special thanks to Julieanne for bringing my words to life through images that stir the soul.

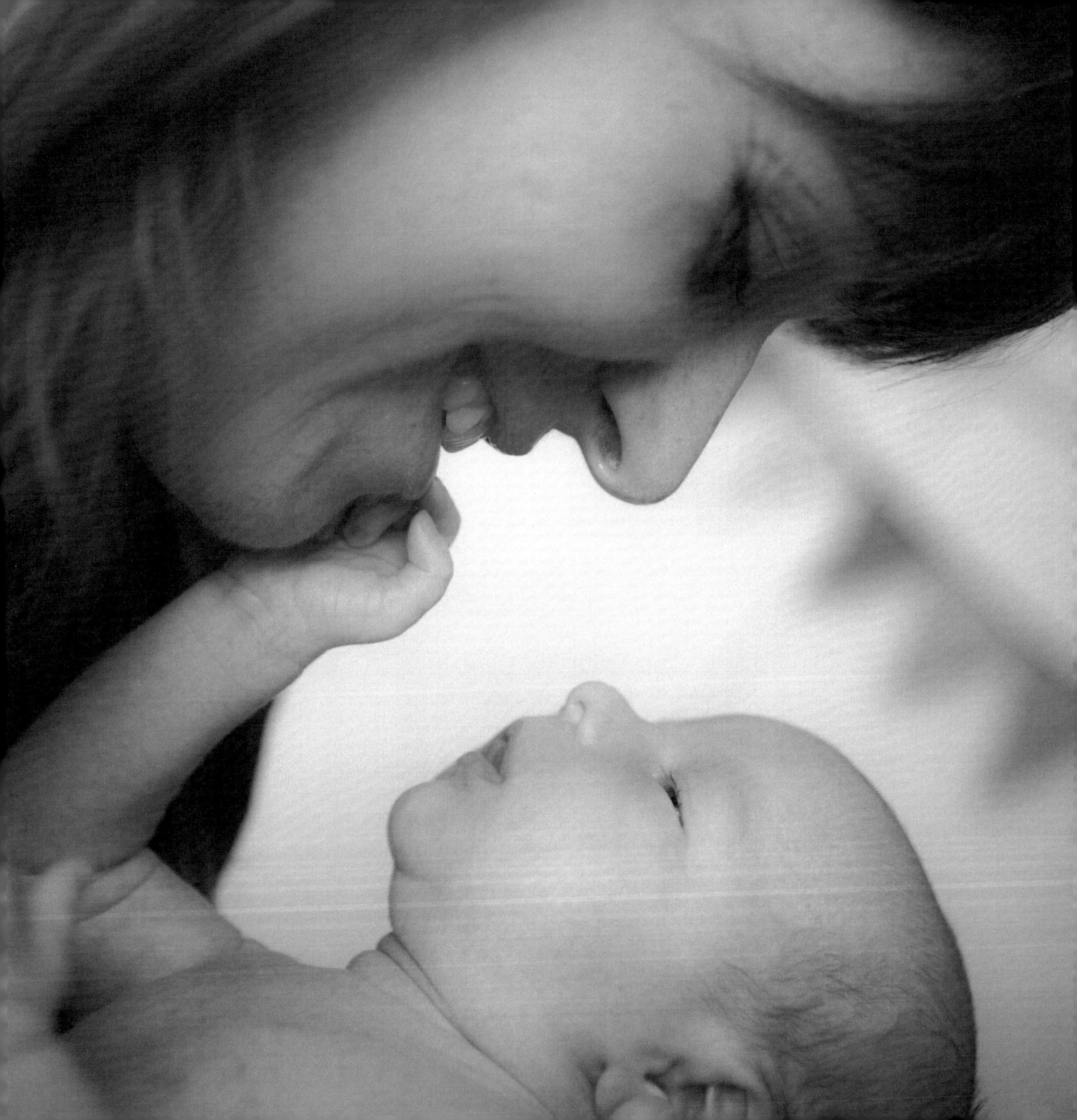

# Forever connected

Through my eyes I see you...

Our hearts connect... forever.

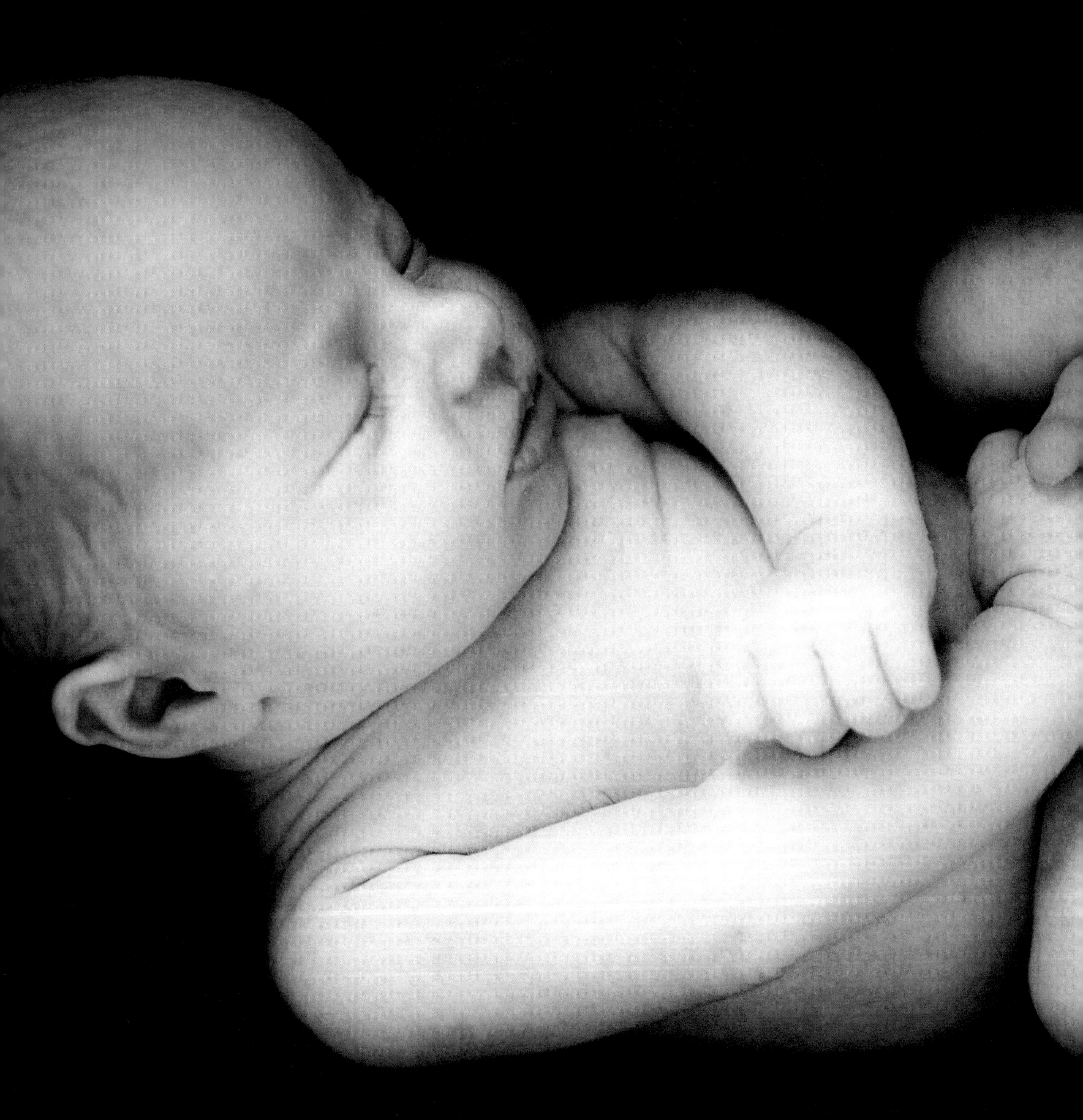

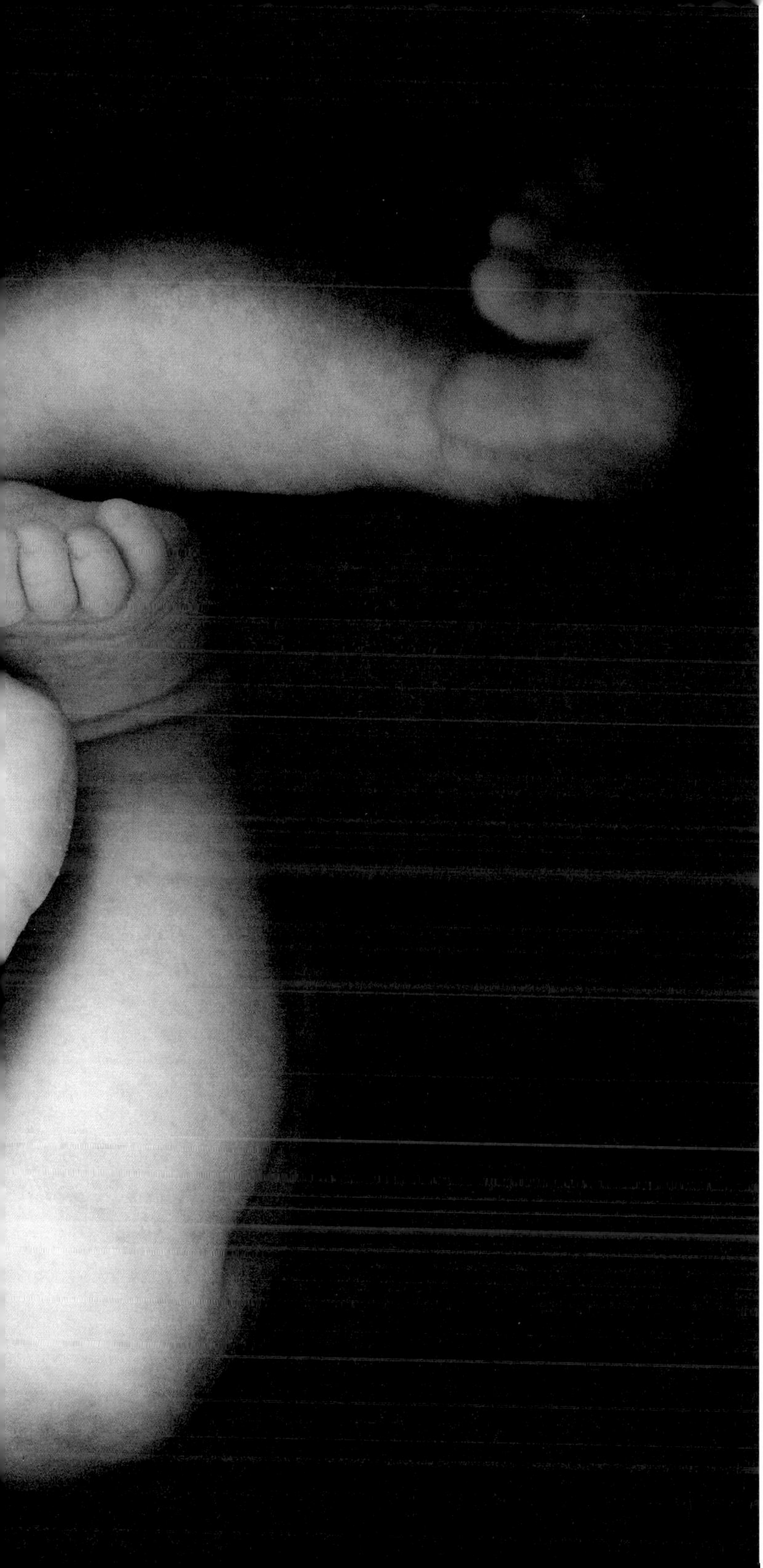

# Here I am

Out from within you.
I take my first breath.
Alone.

Where are you?

This physical
separation is so
daunting.

I cry out to reach you.

Hold me close, often.

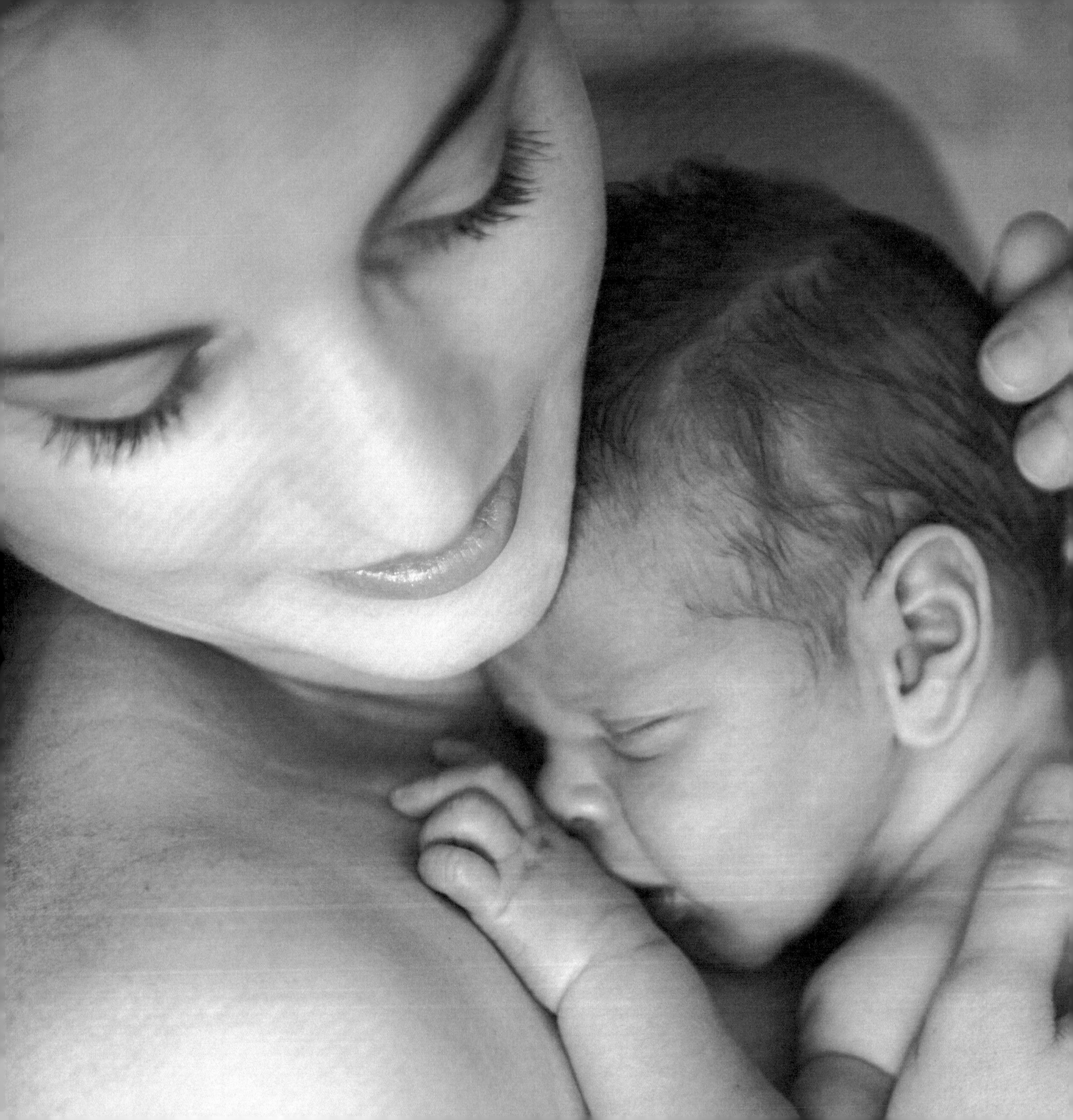

## So big and so small

I'm unsure of this very different space I now live in.

It's so big. I'm so little.

And for the time being, I'm so totally dependent on you... just to survive.

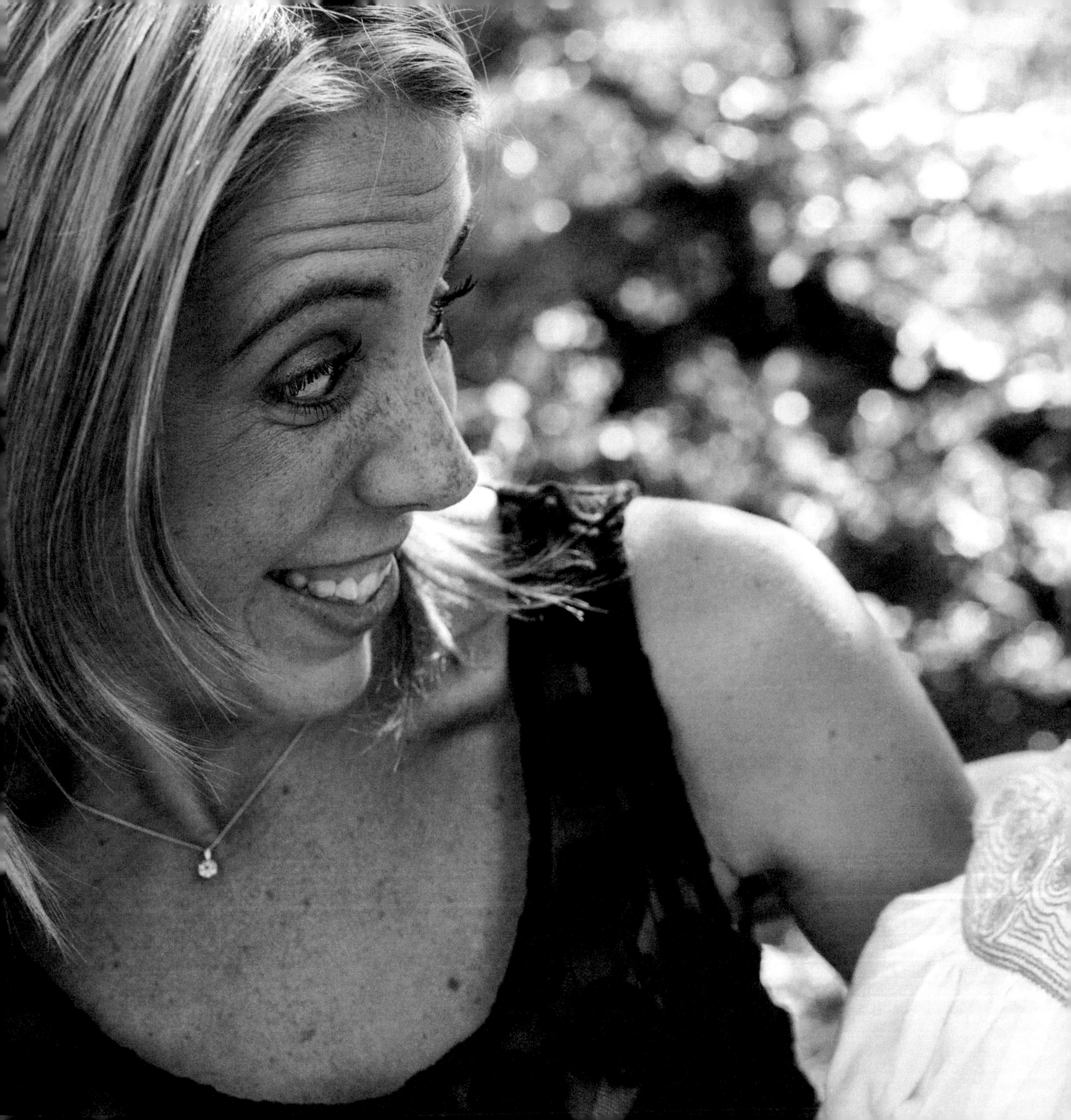

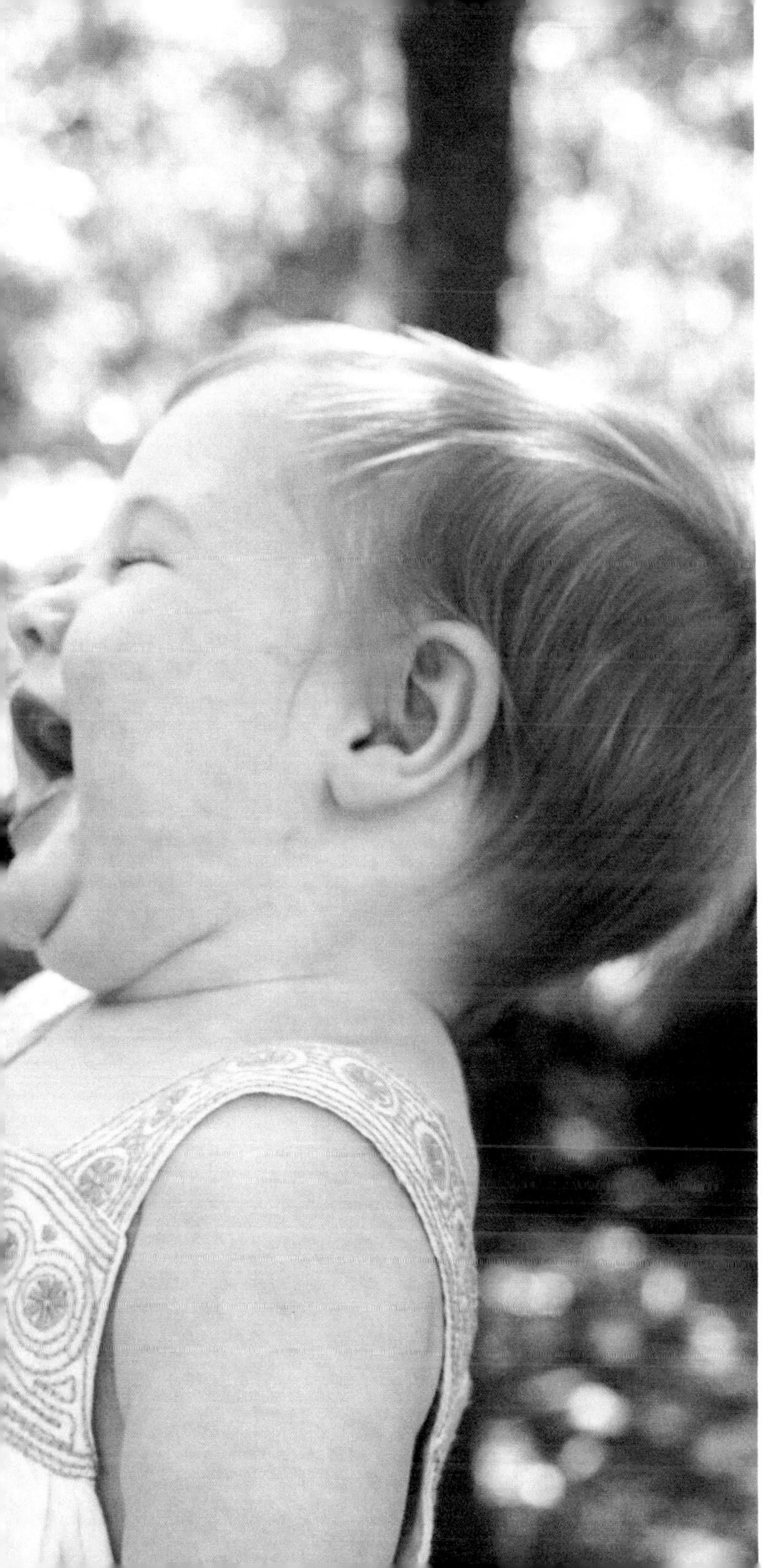

# The energy of us

As if no boundary
between us,
your energy affects
mine.

When you are upset,
angry or anxious,
it unsettles me and
I feel lost and
helpless.

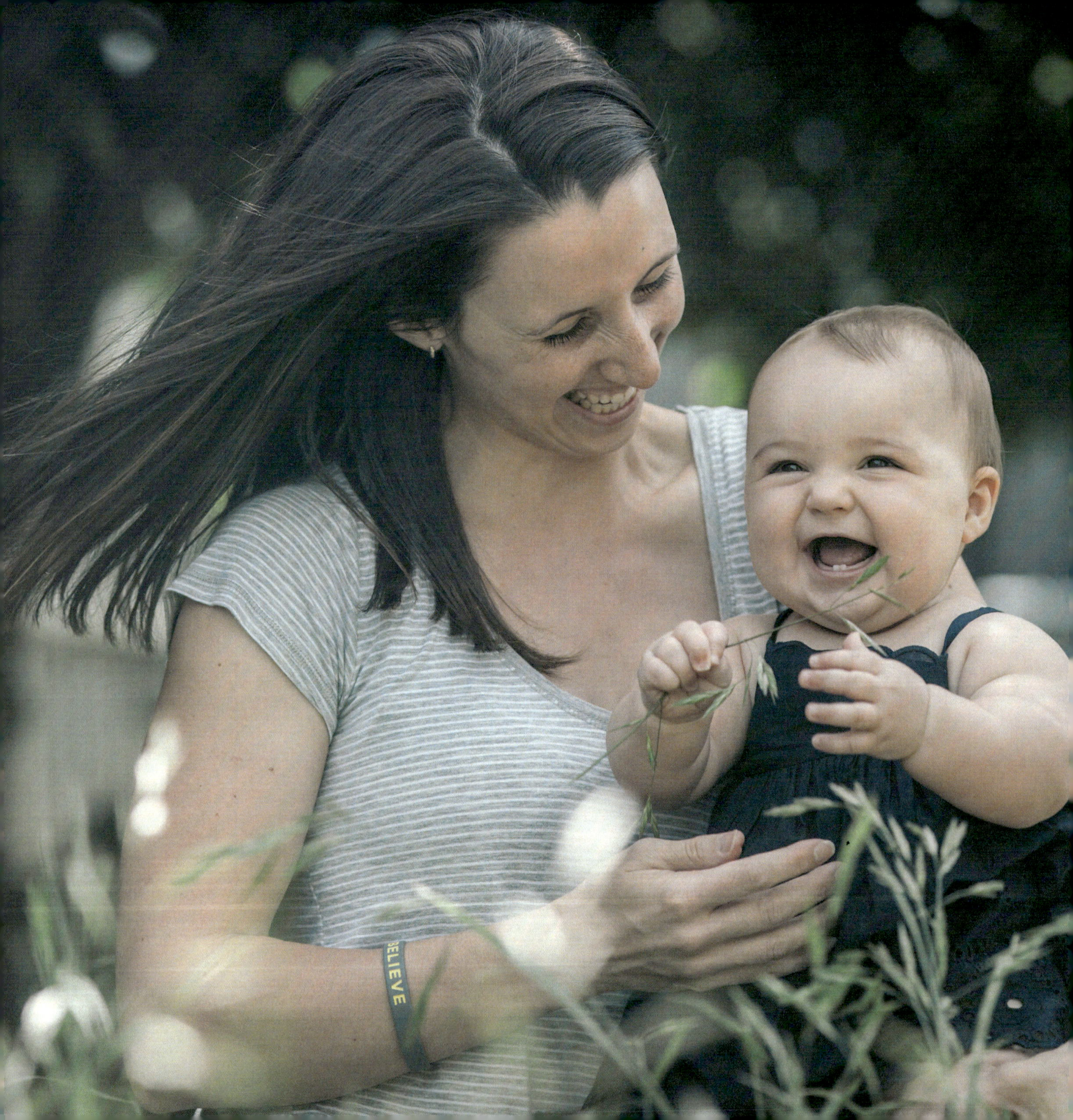
BELIEVE

# Like nothing before

I am capable of eliciting from you such deep love, joy and pride as well as frustration, despair and even anger—like you've never experienced before.

Please be patient with me as I navigate this world and all its wily ways. I'm just a beginner!

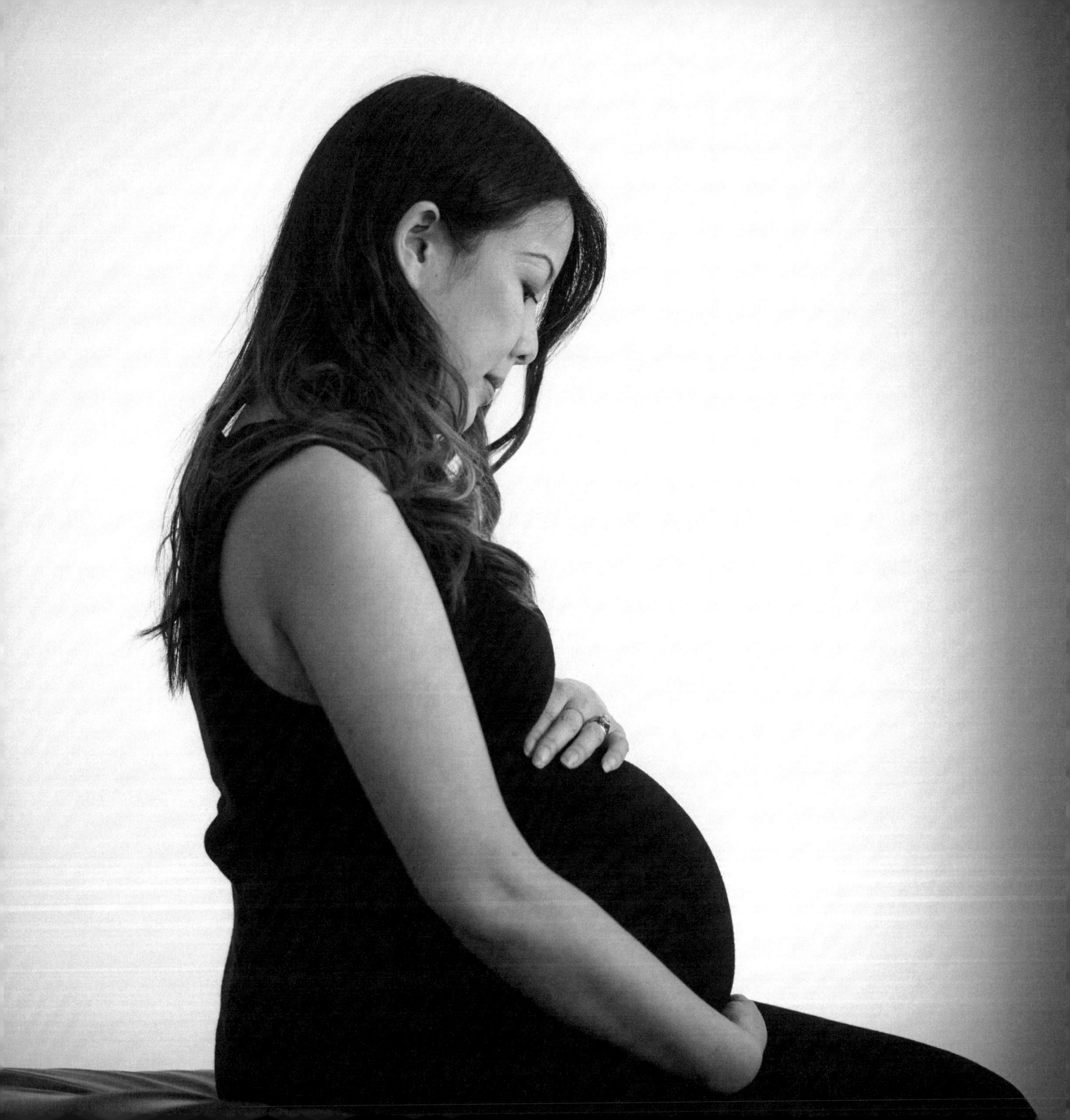

# Finding our way

Not so long ago I was snug in your womb.

Not so long ago, you didn't have me.

So it's okay for both of us to feel a bit wobbly as we adjust to our new way of being and let go of the familiarity and comfort of what we had before.

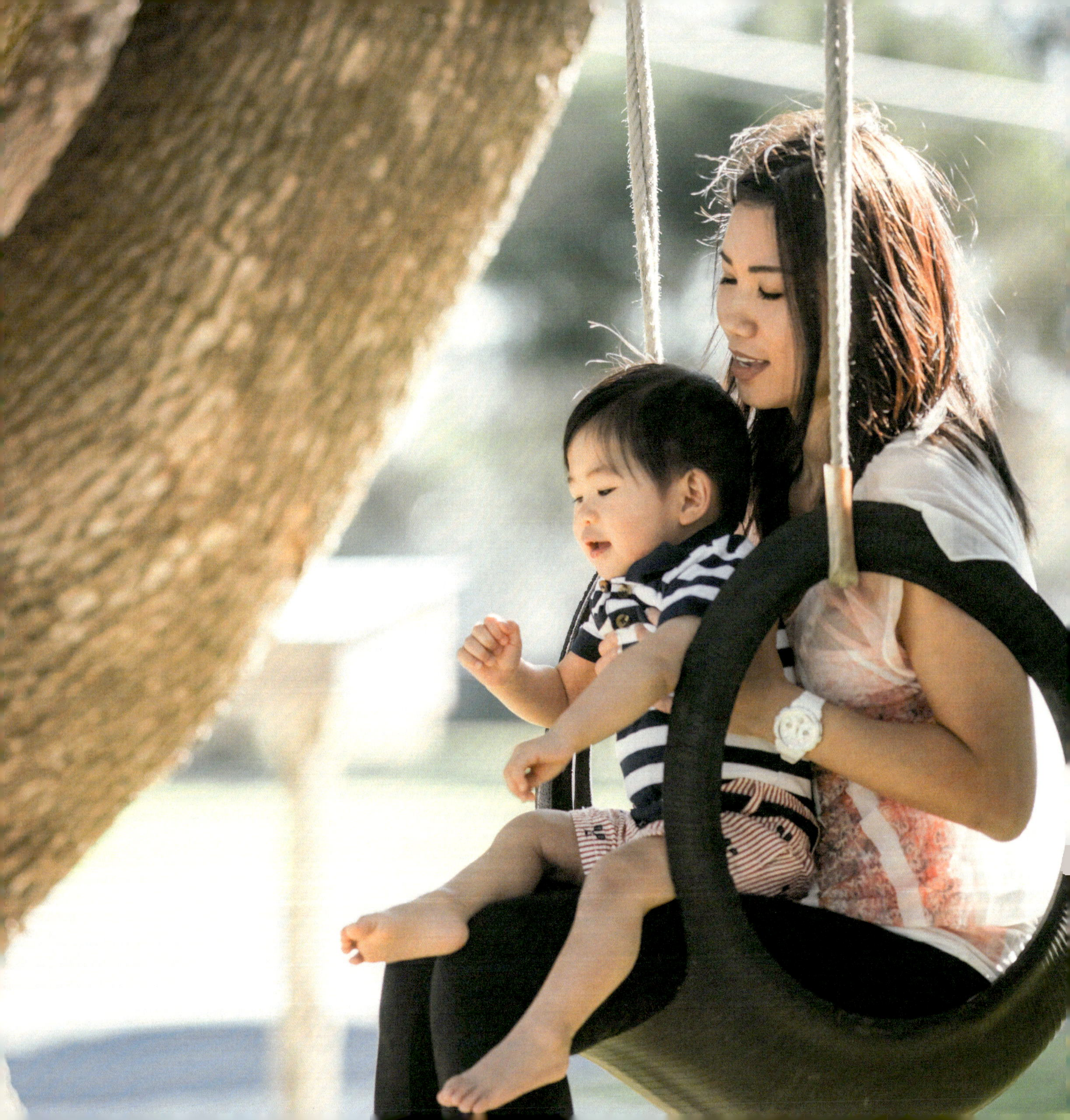

# The time of my life

This is the time of my life when my brain and body grow the most. It may seem so slow to you but for me each day is like climbing a mountain.

With each sleep, my body rests so my brain can start understanding all that is happening around and within me.

It helps me if you relax and slow your time to mine, even though your patience will be tried.

Listen to your tender heart to guide you to a pace that's just fine.

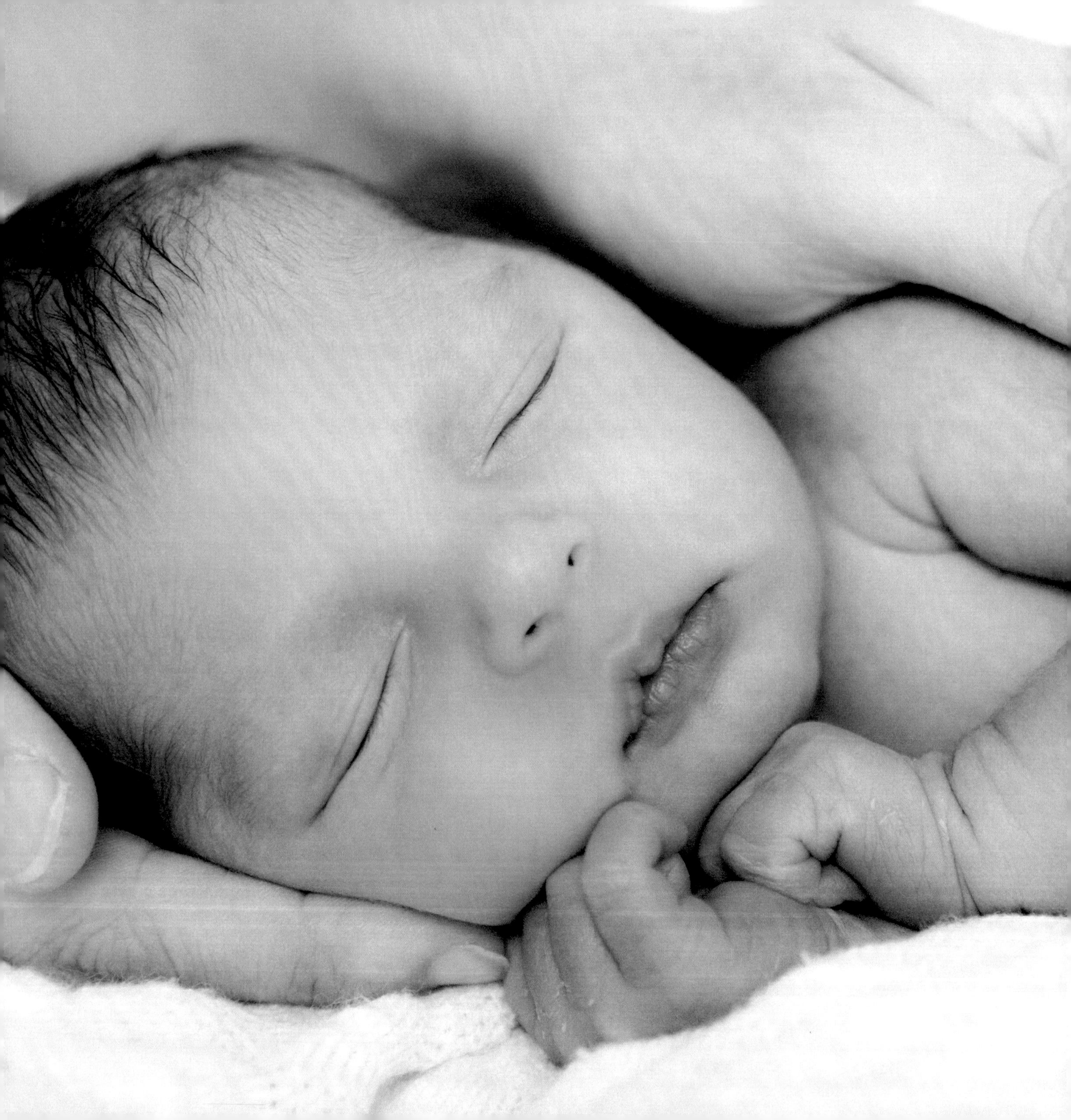

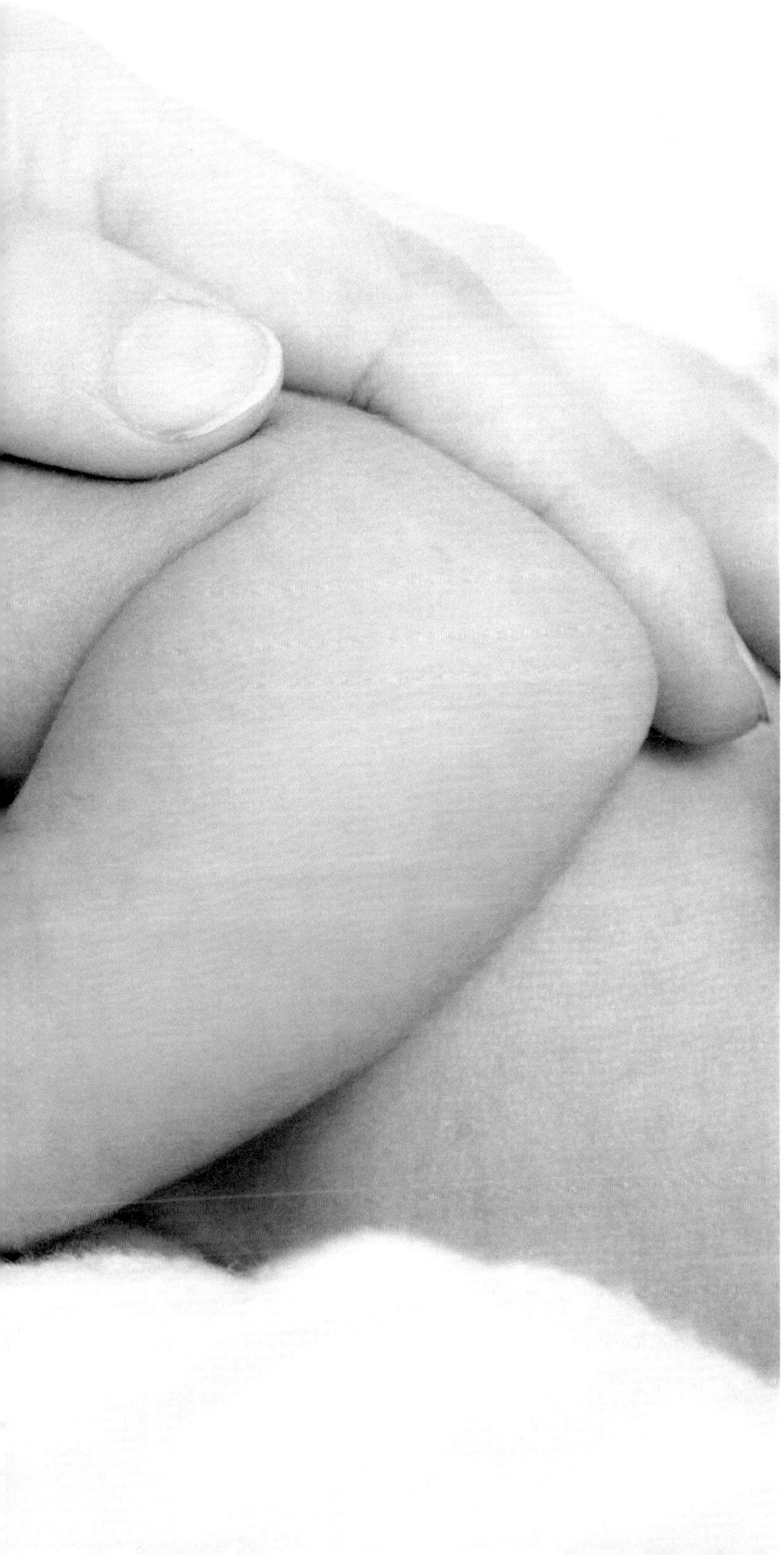

# Thank you for me

For my gift of life, I'll have unconditional love for you.

Even when you don't quite get things right, I'll still love you and trust you—
a treasure to behold.

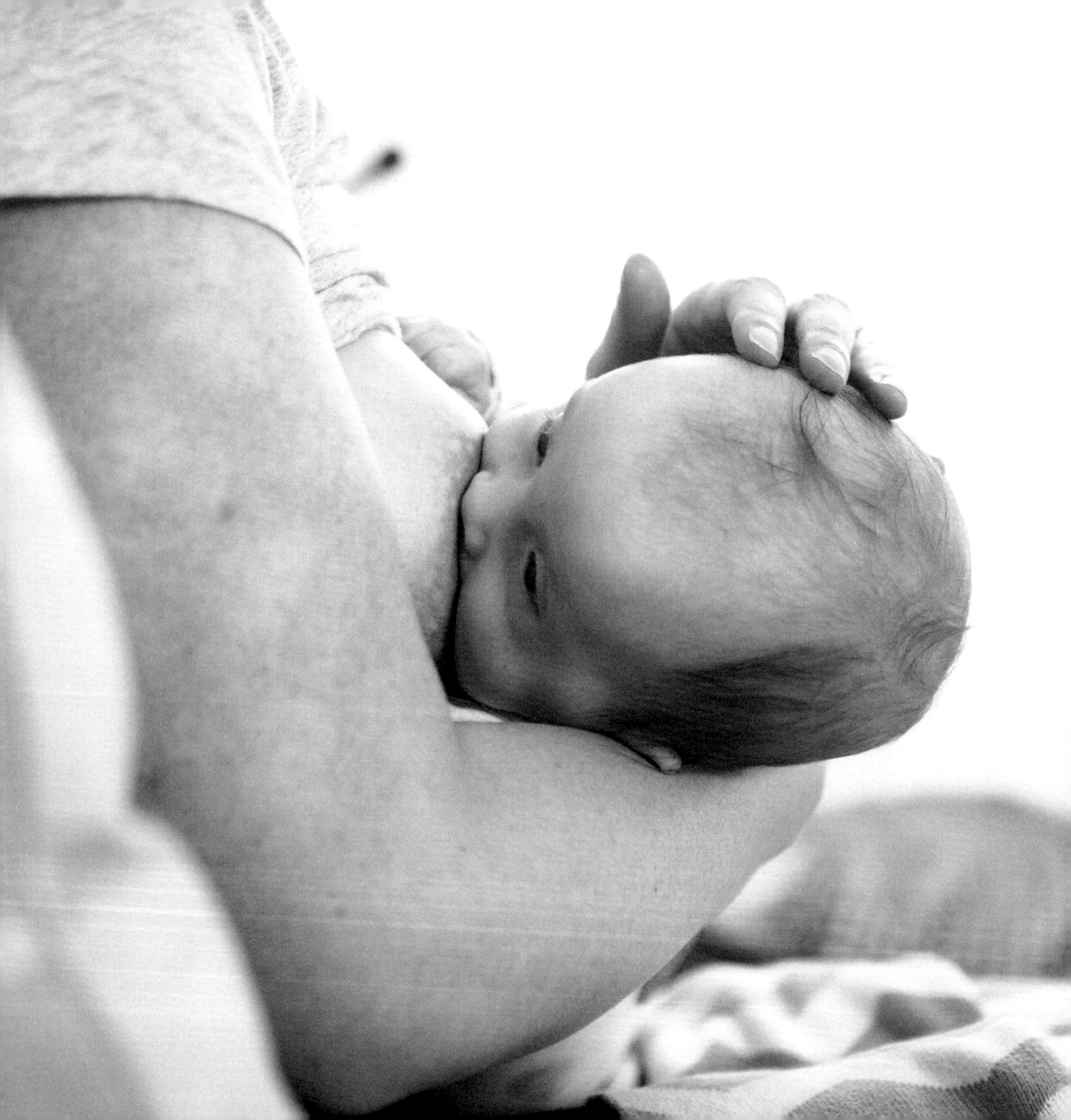

# Your precious milk

I'd love to be breastfed just as nature intended, for your milk with its antibodies, close comfort and bonding. If this is not possible, I can thrive on bottle-fed breast milk or formula.

The milk that makes you happiest is the milk that makes me happiest.

# Tuning-in

In my first few weeks, part of my innate instinct to survive is to make different reflex pre-cry sounds to help you know what I need. Listen very carefully to the subtle differences they make before I get distressed and it's more challenging to work out what I need.

*(Based on Dunstan Baby Language and the work of Dunstan Baby Institute researchers)*

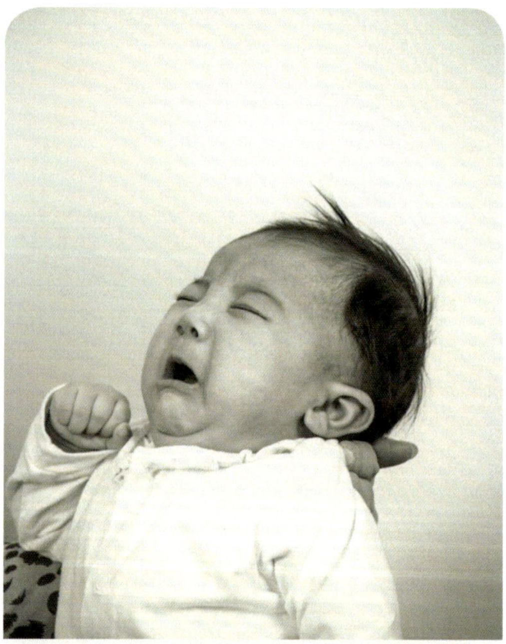

'Neh' is loud and rhythmic and means I'm hungry.

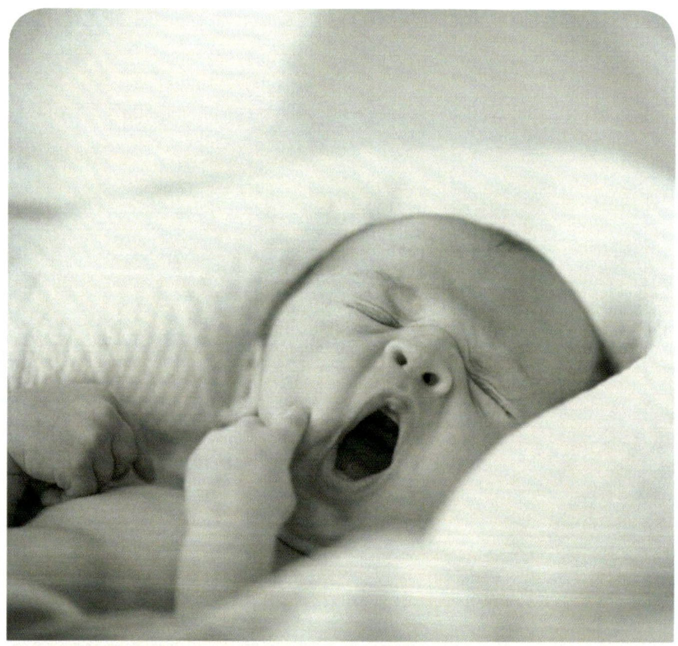

'Owh' is a yawn reflex and means I'm sleepy.

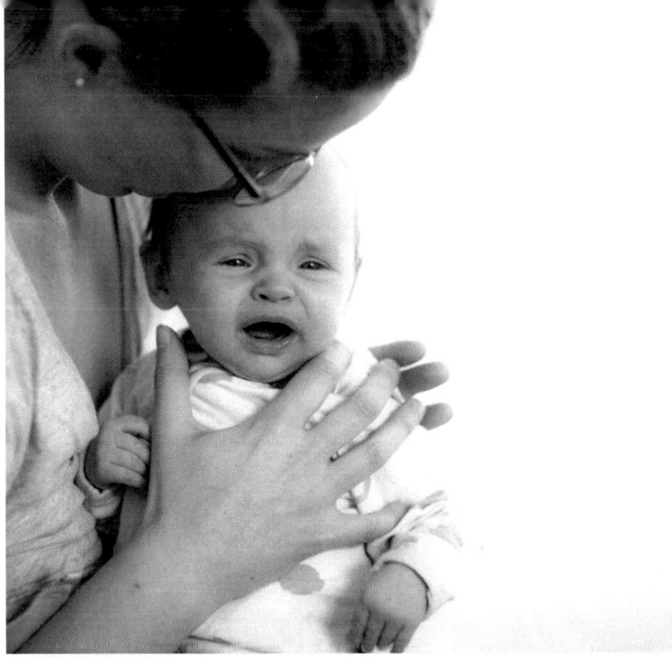

'Eh ehhhh' means I need to burp. Sit me up or lift me up against your shoulder to help the wind out.

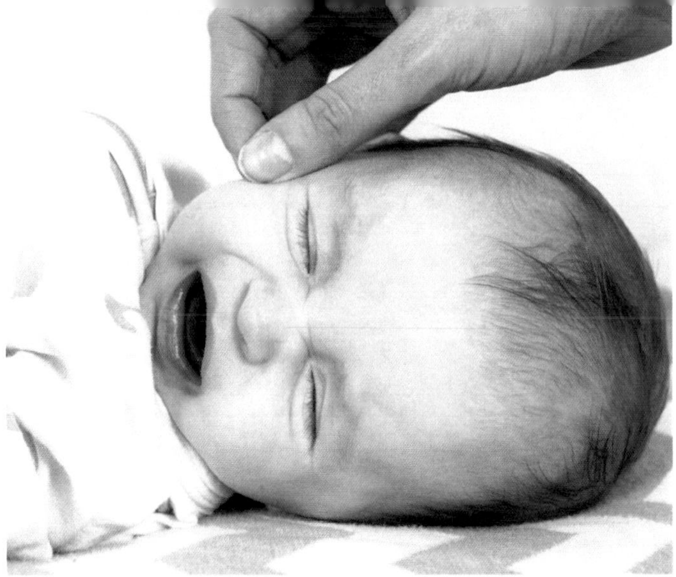

'Eair' means lower gas. My face and body squirm and my legs pull up or push out. Lift me up and nurse me through this most uncomfortable time 'til my wind works its way through my body.

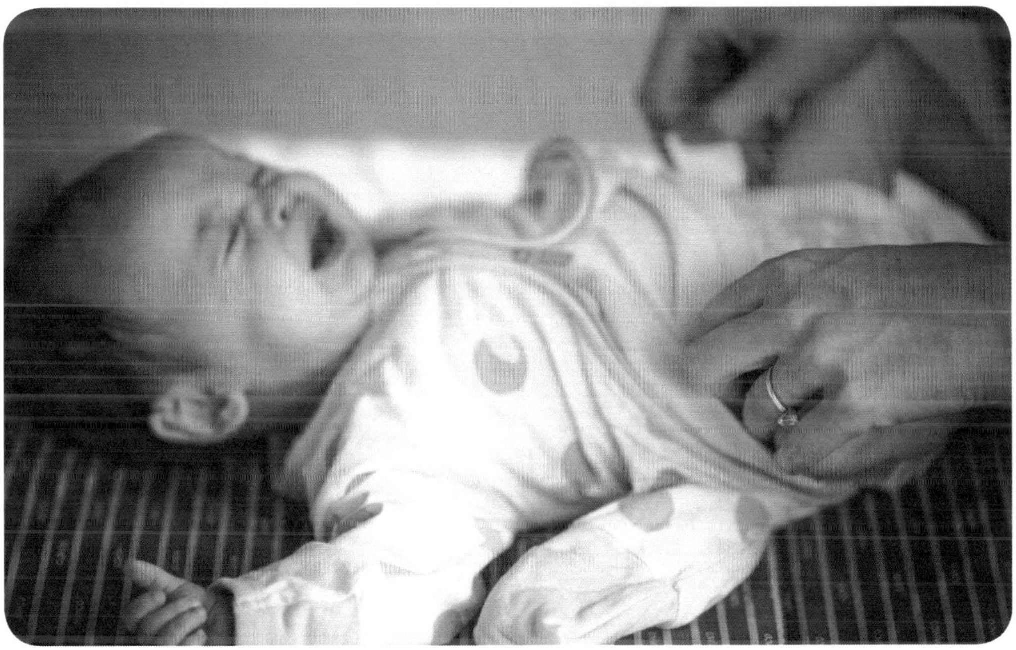

'Heh' means I'm uncomfortable and need something like a nappy change or position change.

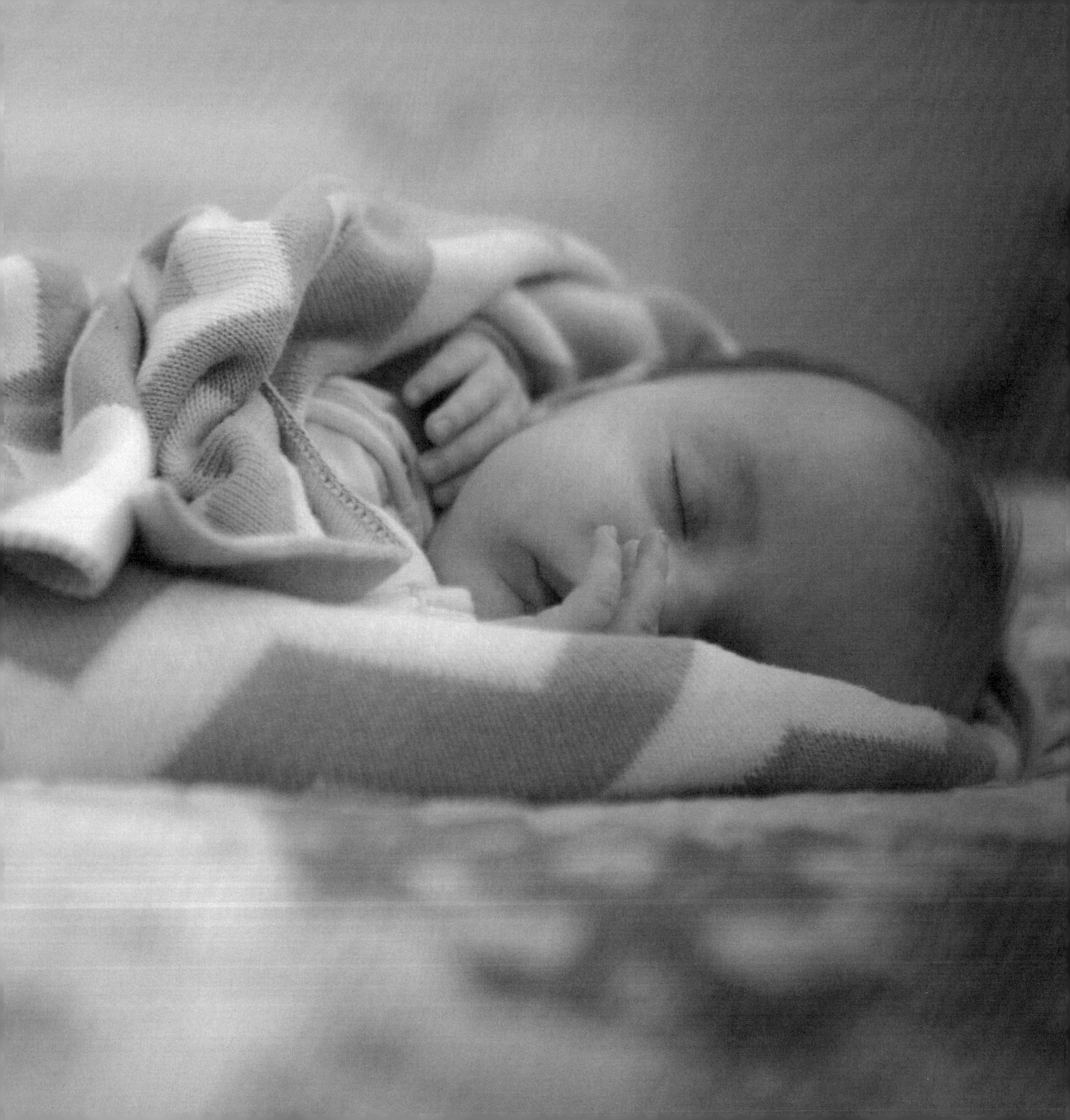

# Sleeping like a baby

I sleep peacefully on a cloud full of your love and affection.

My short cycle of sleep, wake, feed, interact and play—will start to lengthen in time.

A darkened room helps my body release chemicals that relax and help me sleep.

If I can't get myself to sleep or become overtired, I'll cry to let you know I need your help.

Respond to me soon so I don't get so distressed and exhausted that I drop off to sleep.

You may think I've self-soothed, but that's beyond my ability at this stage.

I need to know you will come to me when I cry.

A cuddle and your calm assurance until I've settled is usually all it takes.

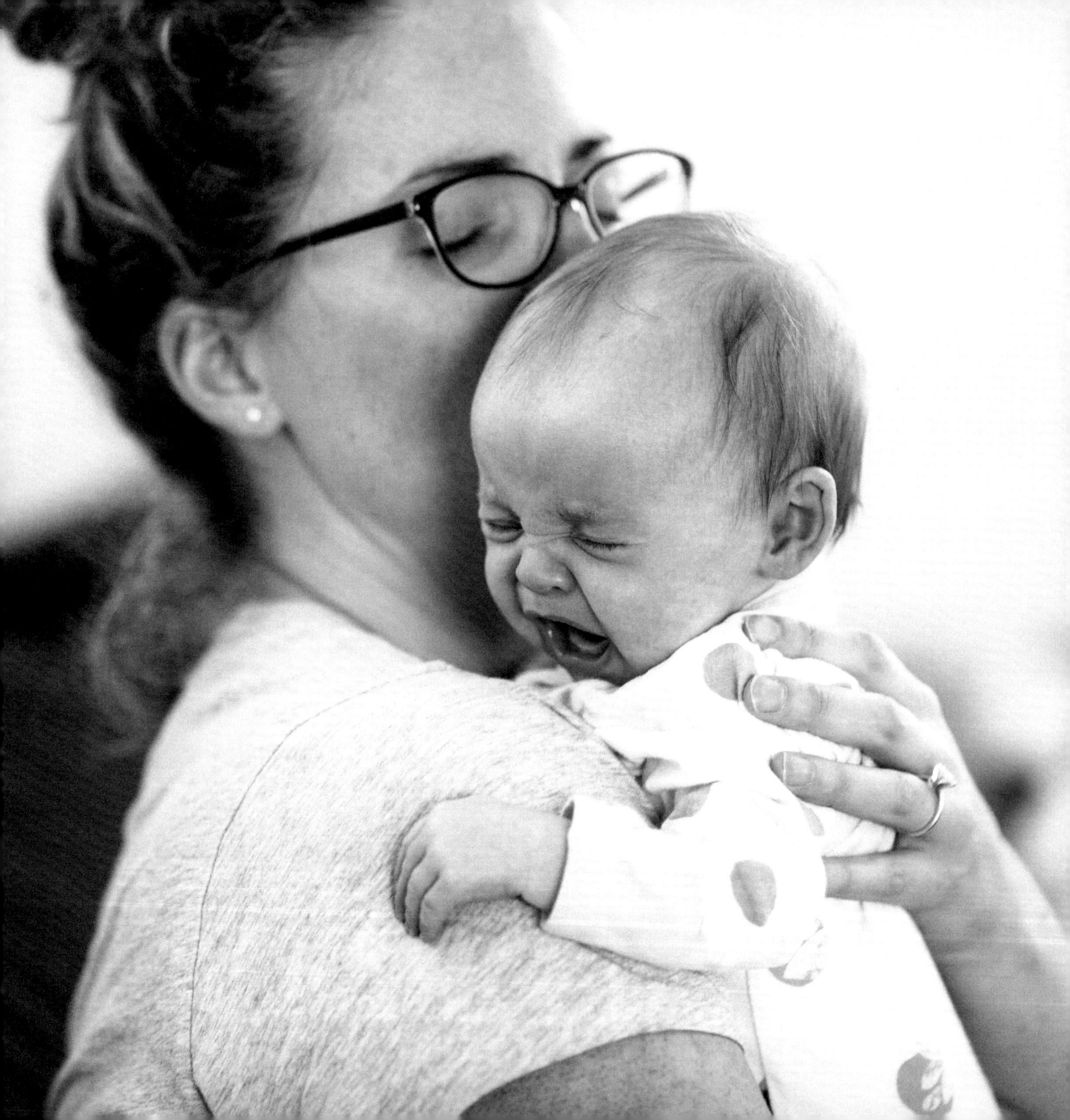

# Crying for no reason

Should I cry for apparently no reason,
or become quite distressed, your close comfort
and care is what I need most.

Perhaps I'm still to adjust my daily rhythm
to yours and this world's night and day.

You will not spoil me by holding or comforting me.

It actually works the opposite.

Your loving care helps soothe me through my
bumpy bits, something I can't do for myself
for quite some time.

Give me some routine so I come to know what
you want from me.

If you think something might be wrong,
don't hesitate to get help.

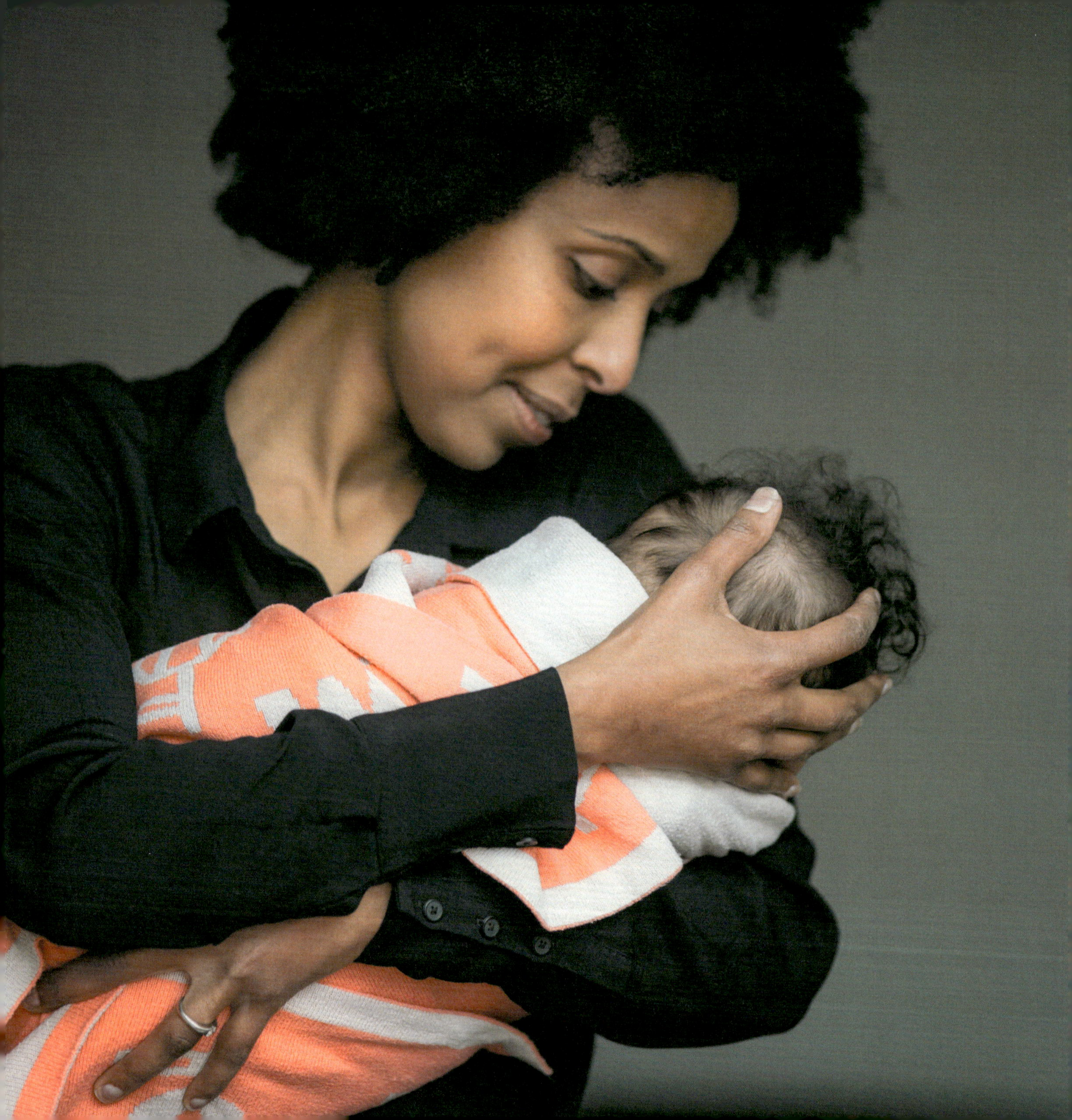

# From crying to calm

Once you've attended to my needs yet still I cry, this may help:

Swaddle me snuggly with my arms tucked in.

Side-lie me across your arm slightly face down.

"Sshhh" quite loudly near my ear.

Swing or jiggle my head gently as it rests in your hand.

Let me suck on a pacifier.

This mimicking my time in your womb provides familiarity that's quite settling for me.

(See Dr Harvey Karp for more detail)

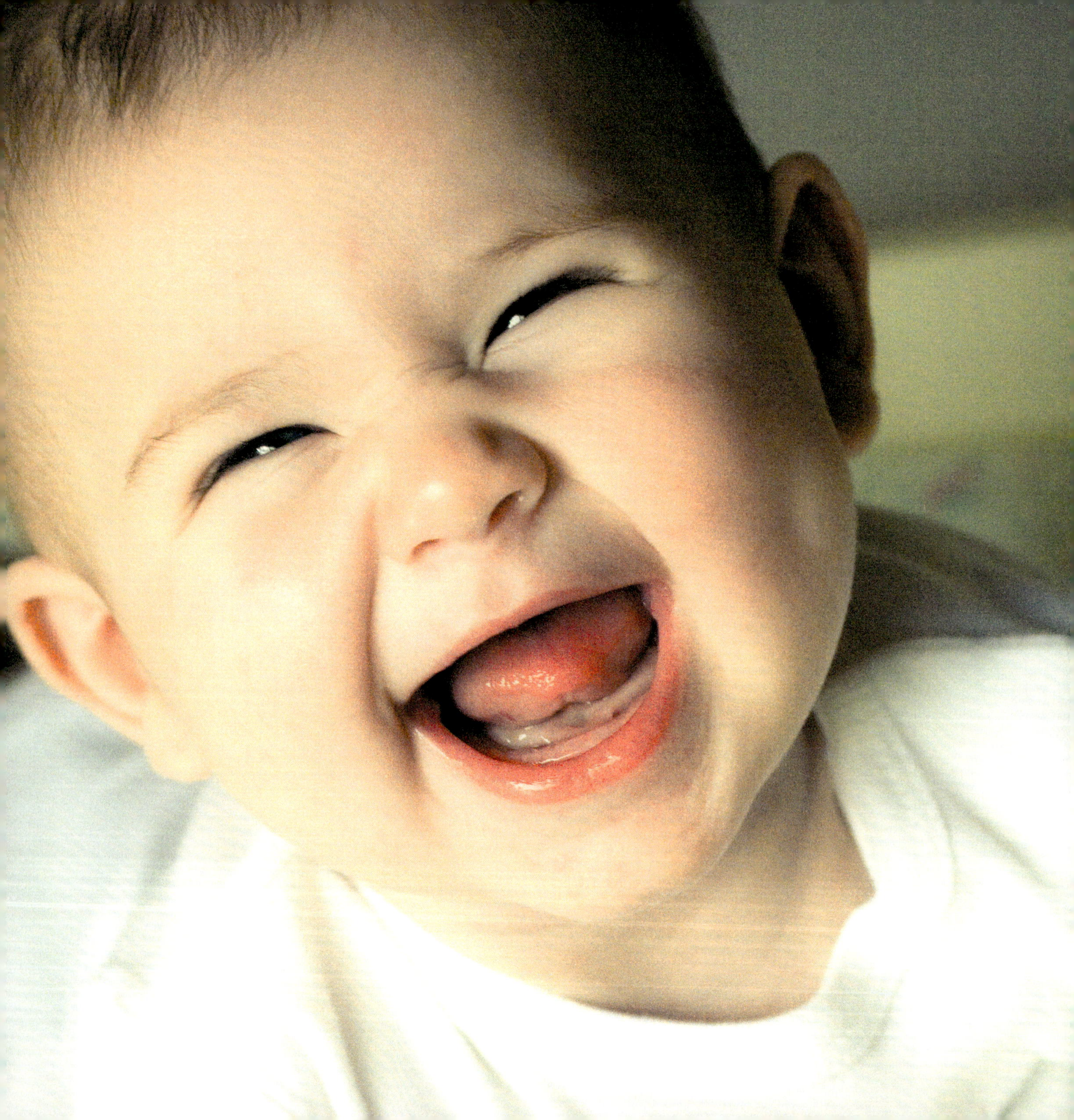

# Awakening to me

With each breath every cell in my body awakens to the individual I am becoming.

I am of you but not you. I am like you but will never become you.

Excuse me while I'm fascinated with myself and my needs are my total focus.

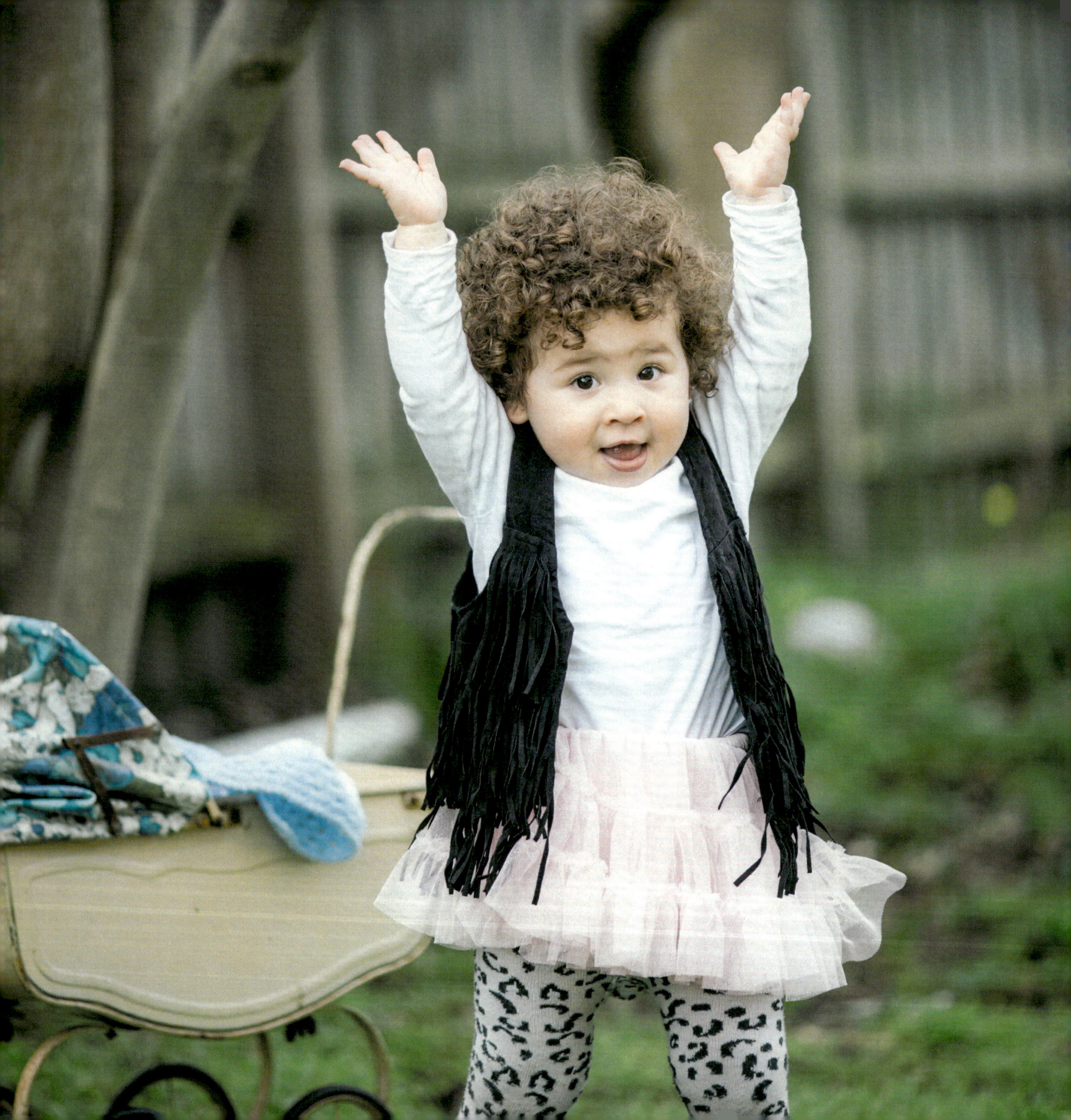

Such an adventure to discover ME!

And with your help, I'll soon discover others and the world beyond me.

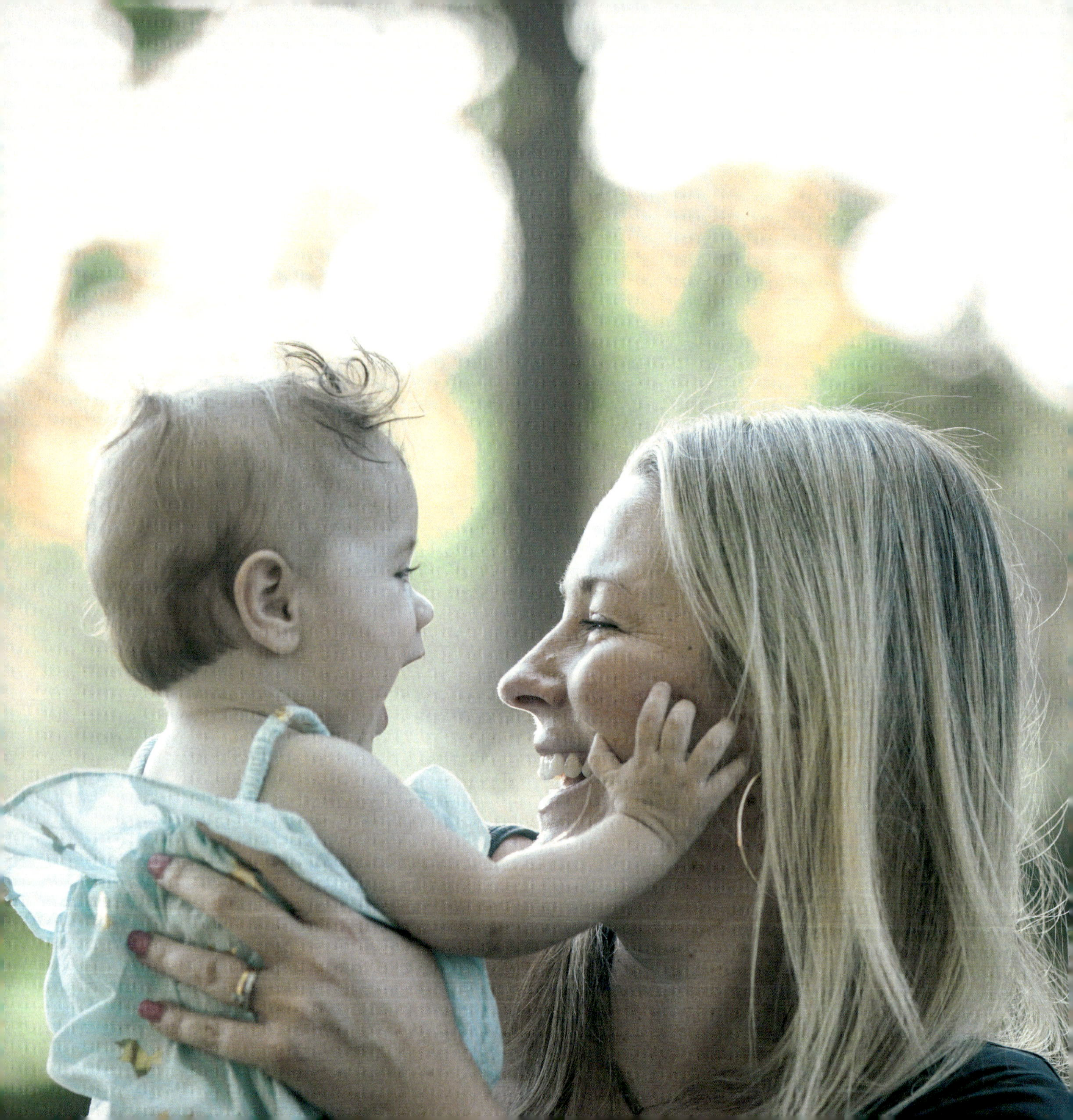

# The eyes have it

Look into my eyes to let me know I have your full attention and connect with me deeply at a heart level.

This will foster good communication between us... for the rest of our lives... and with others.

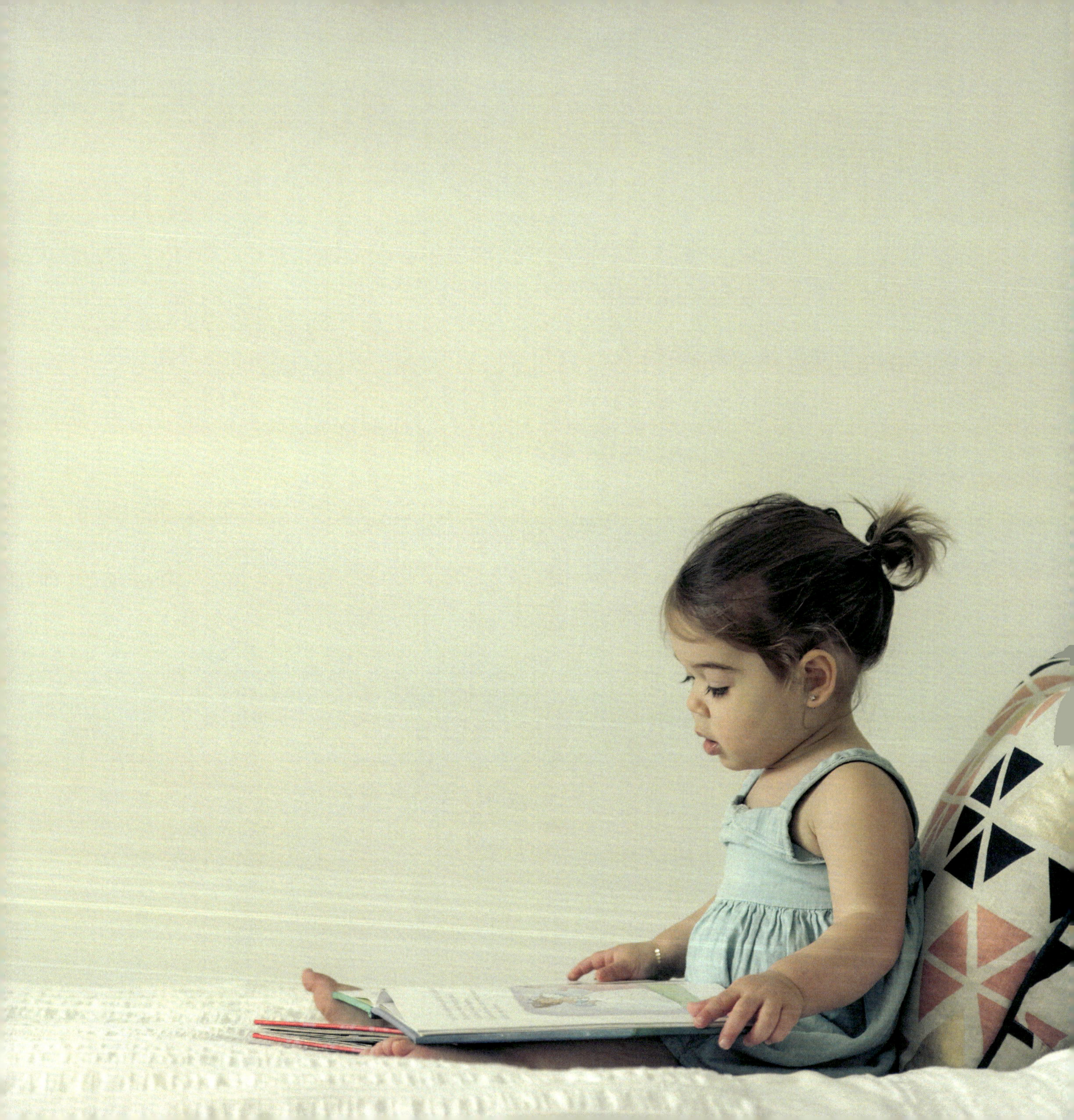

# Safe enough, free to learn

When you and my surroundings are calm and predictable, I feel safe enough to turn my attention away from you and begin to learn new things.

When my surroundings are otherwise, my energy and focus turns to survival and learning can be delayed or not come at all.

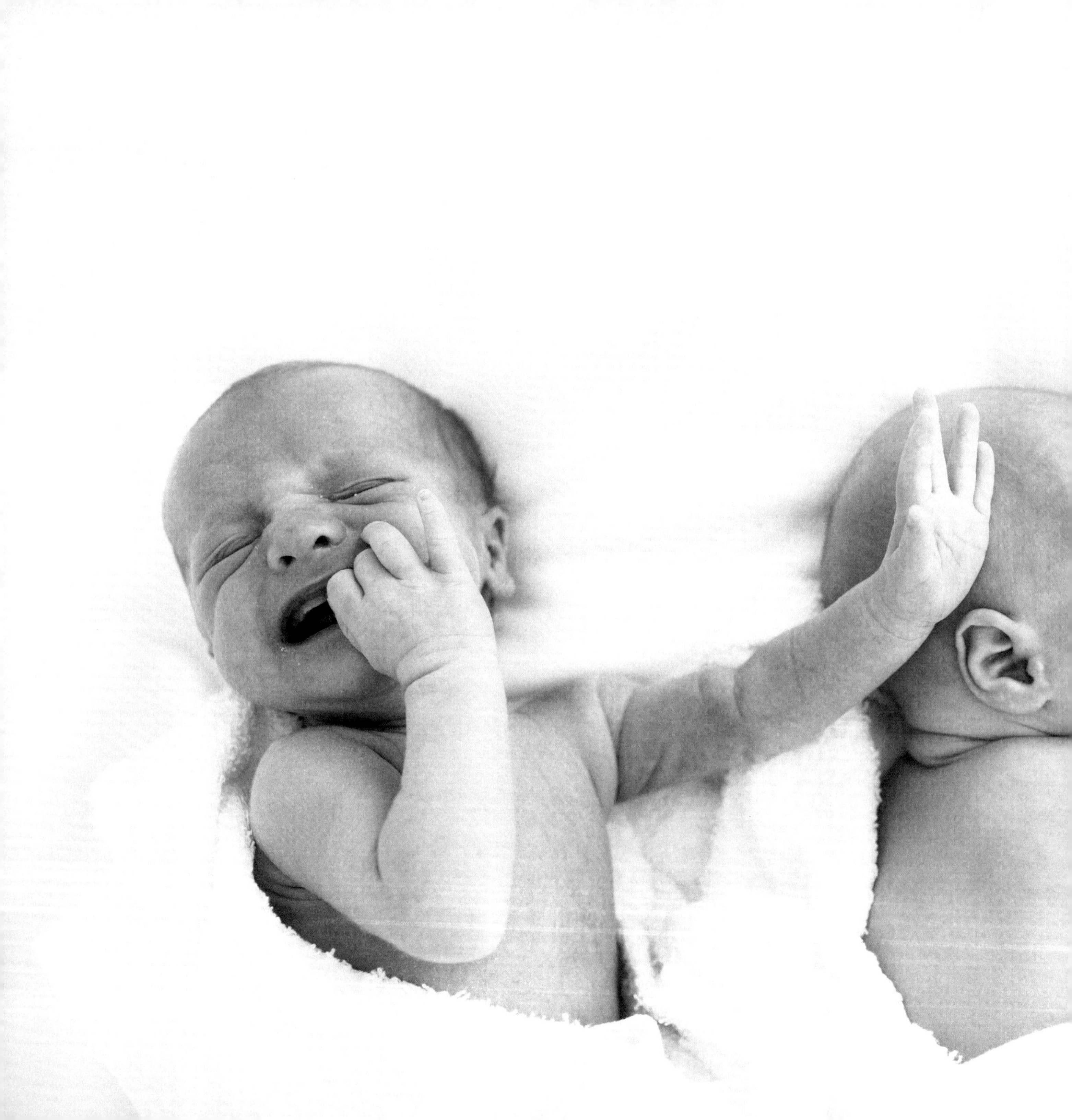

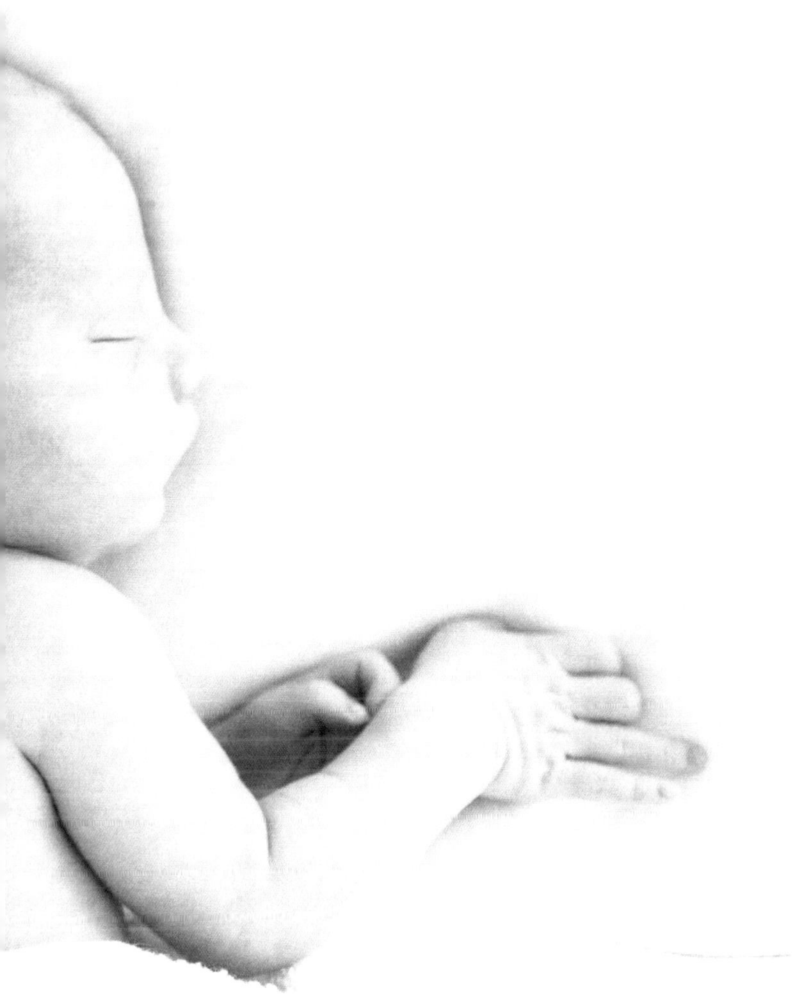

# Good one day, unsettled the next

From one day to the next I can behave in different and unpredictable ways.

I am not doing this on purpose or in any way trying to annoy you.

I could be having a growth spurt or a reaction to something in my environment.

Accept each day as it comes.

Aim for progression rather than perfection to make things easier for both of us.

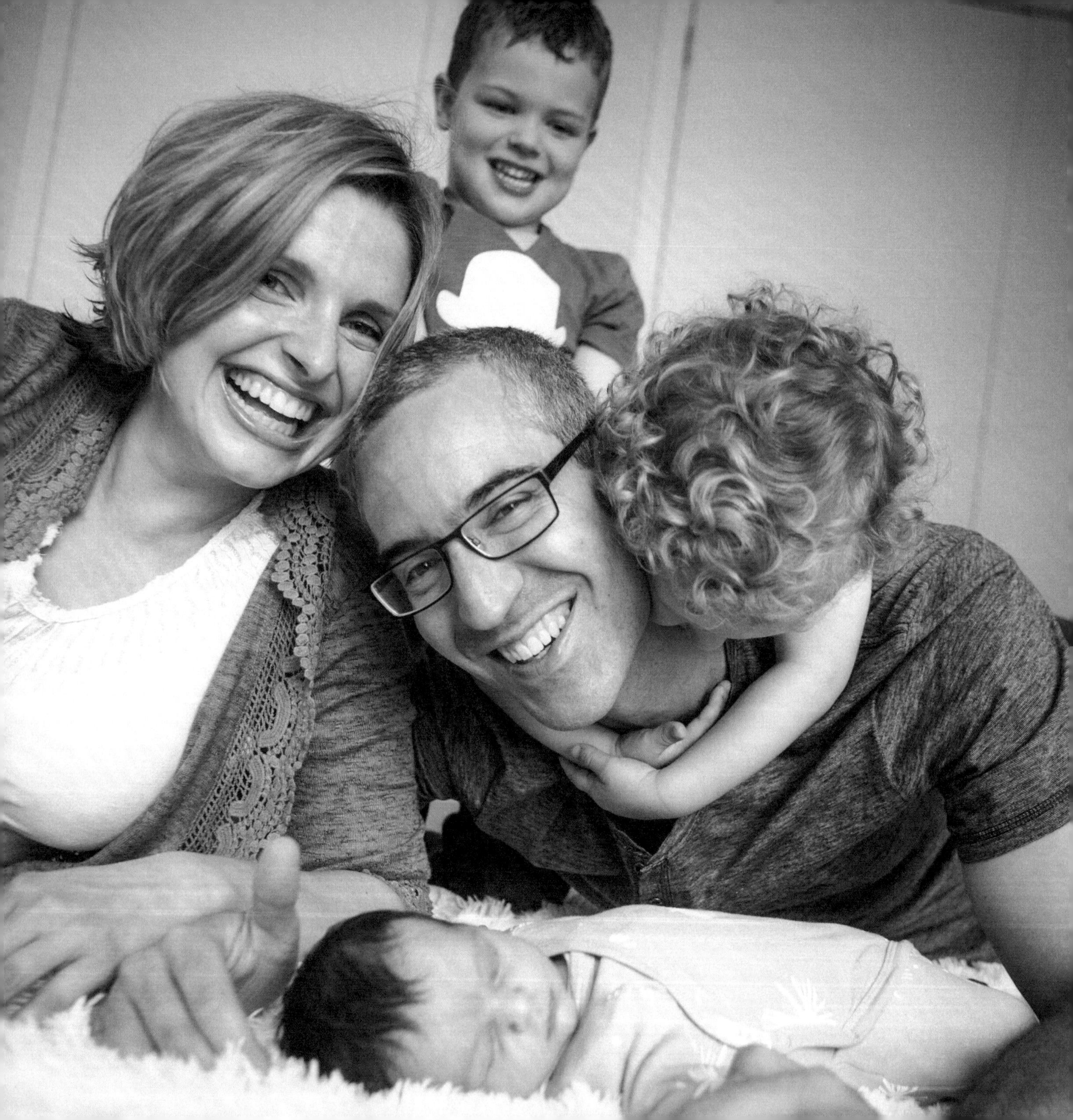

# Attention, affection and stimulation

Fun, cuddles, laughter and love help my brain develop healthily.

Get down and play with me regularly to deepen our bond and connection.

With these beautiful memories deposited into my 'emotional bank', I will come to withstand being away from you by 'drawing on it' to get me through until we're reunited.

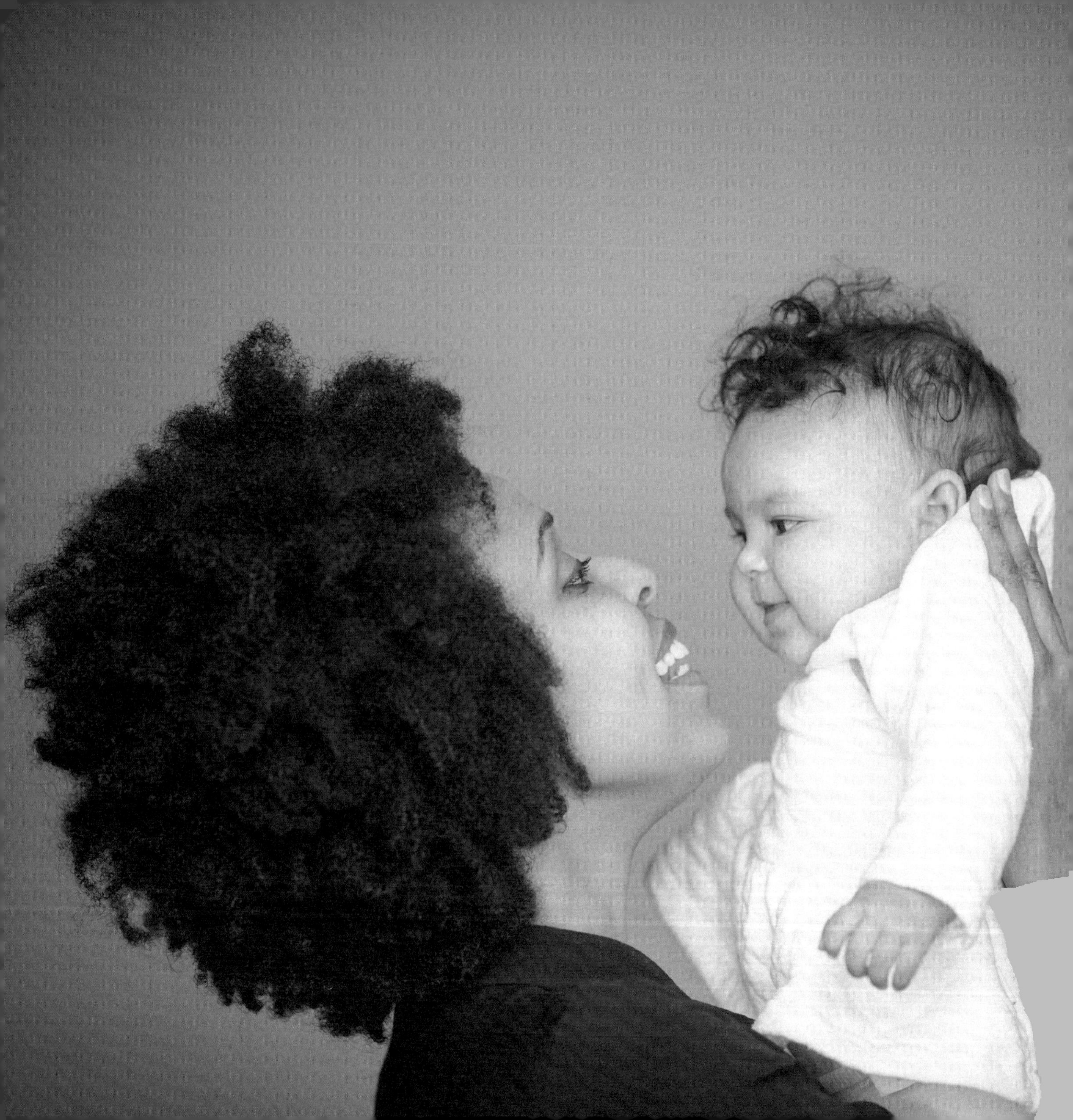

# The music of your voice

When we're up close, I feel the vibration of your words and the language I'll soon speak.

Enrich my being with the beautiful music that kind words chime. And read aloud or sing to me so I hear the songs of others, both imaginary and real.

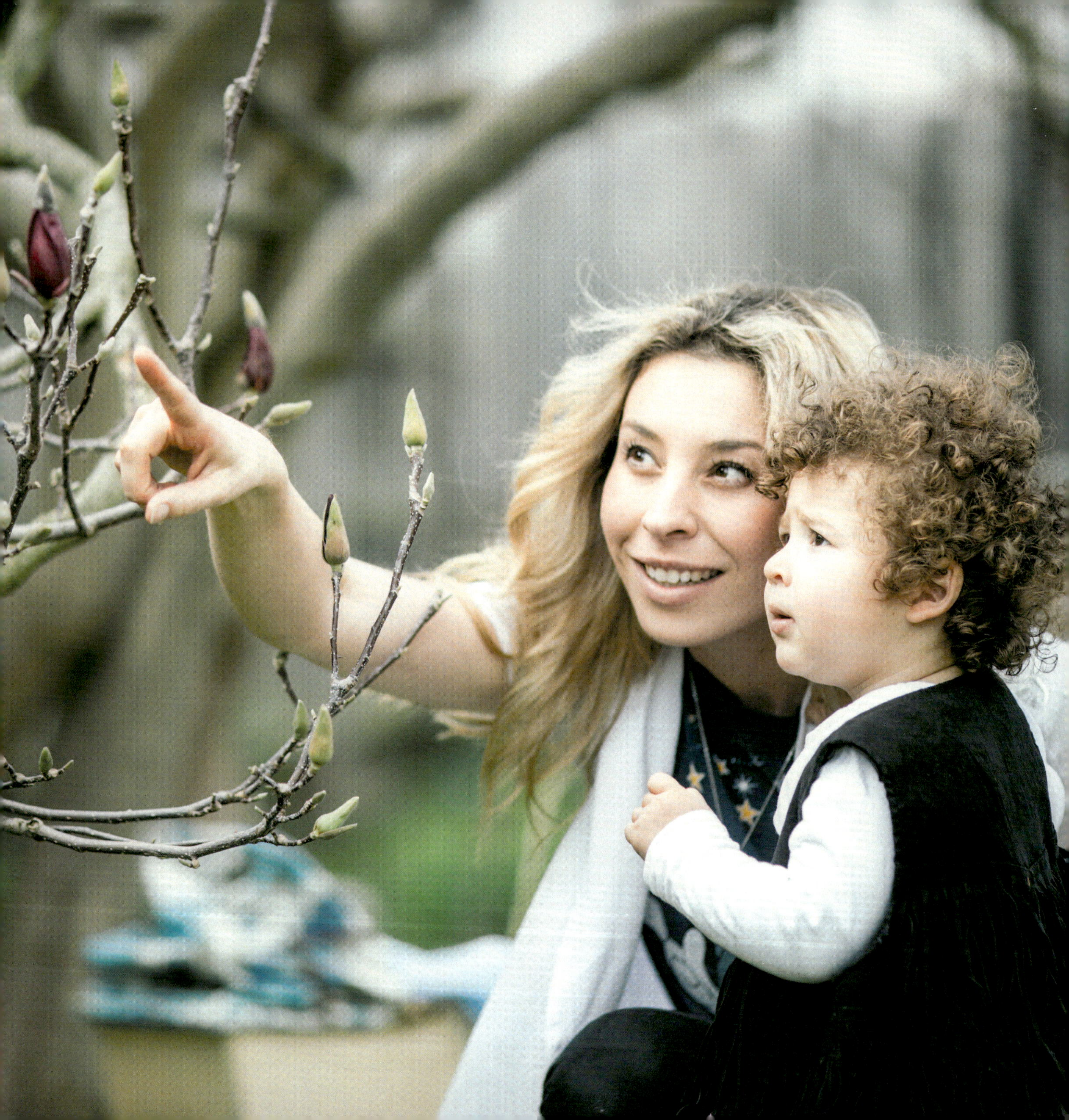

# Always my mother

I want and need you to be my mother—different to being a friend.

I will make my own friends in time, just like you have done. Please be my mother, so it's not confusing for you or me.

We can have lots of fun and share very special times together—as mother and child, just the way it's meant to be.

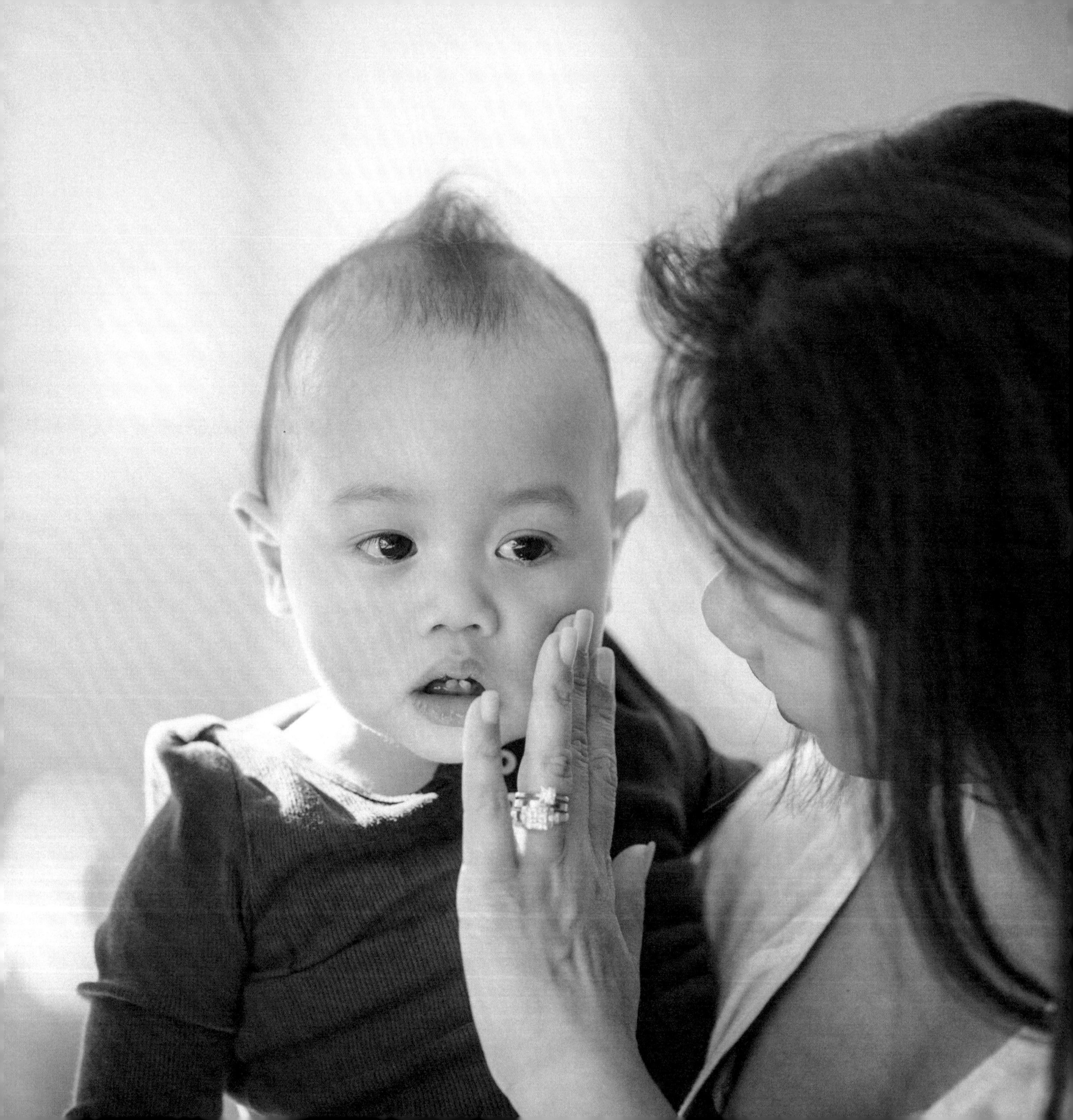

# The power of you

When you attend to my needs with your loving care, I learn to trust you... and others.

What you do, I will copy.

How you treat me is how I'll start to treat others.

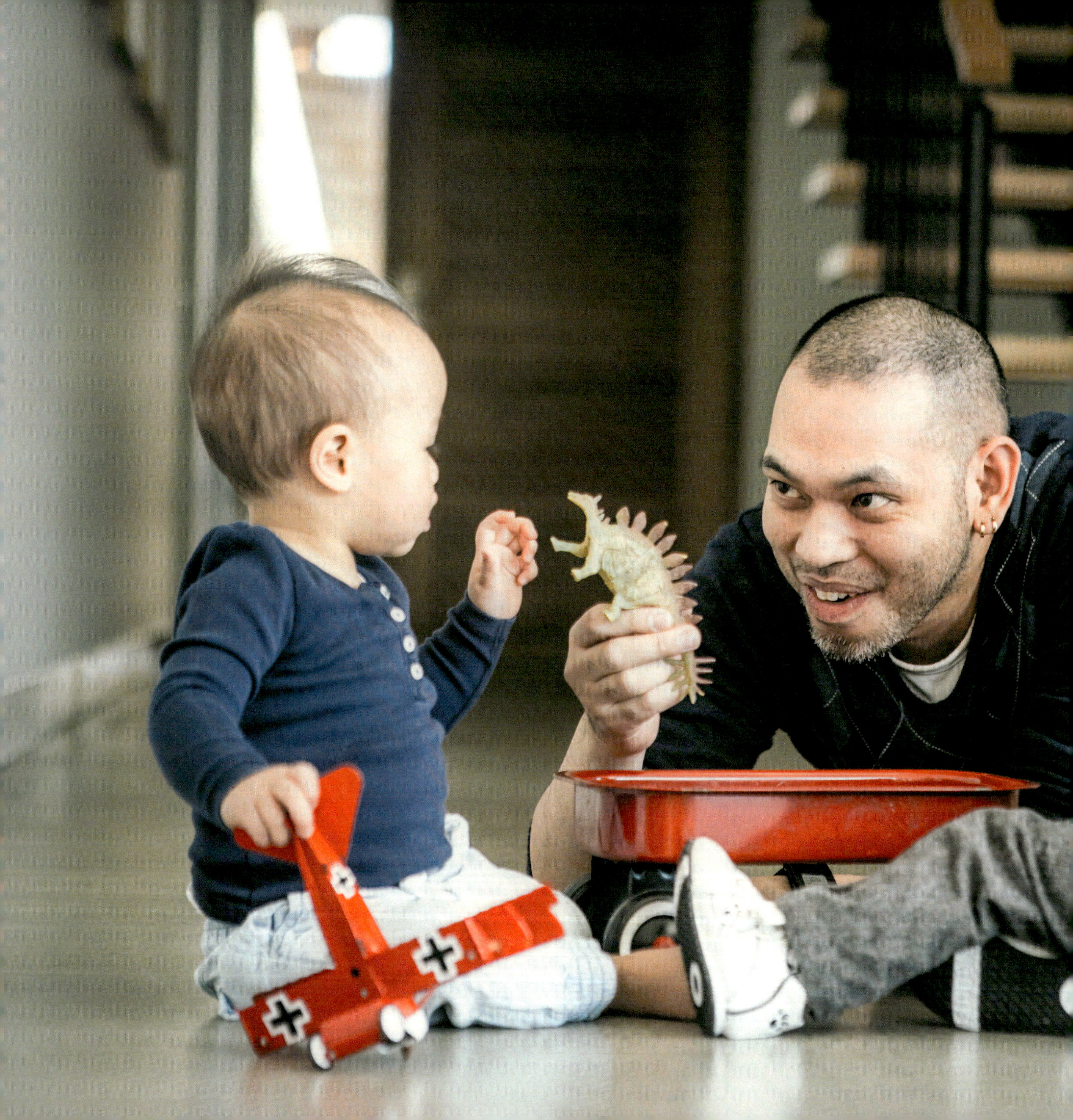

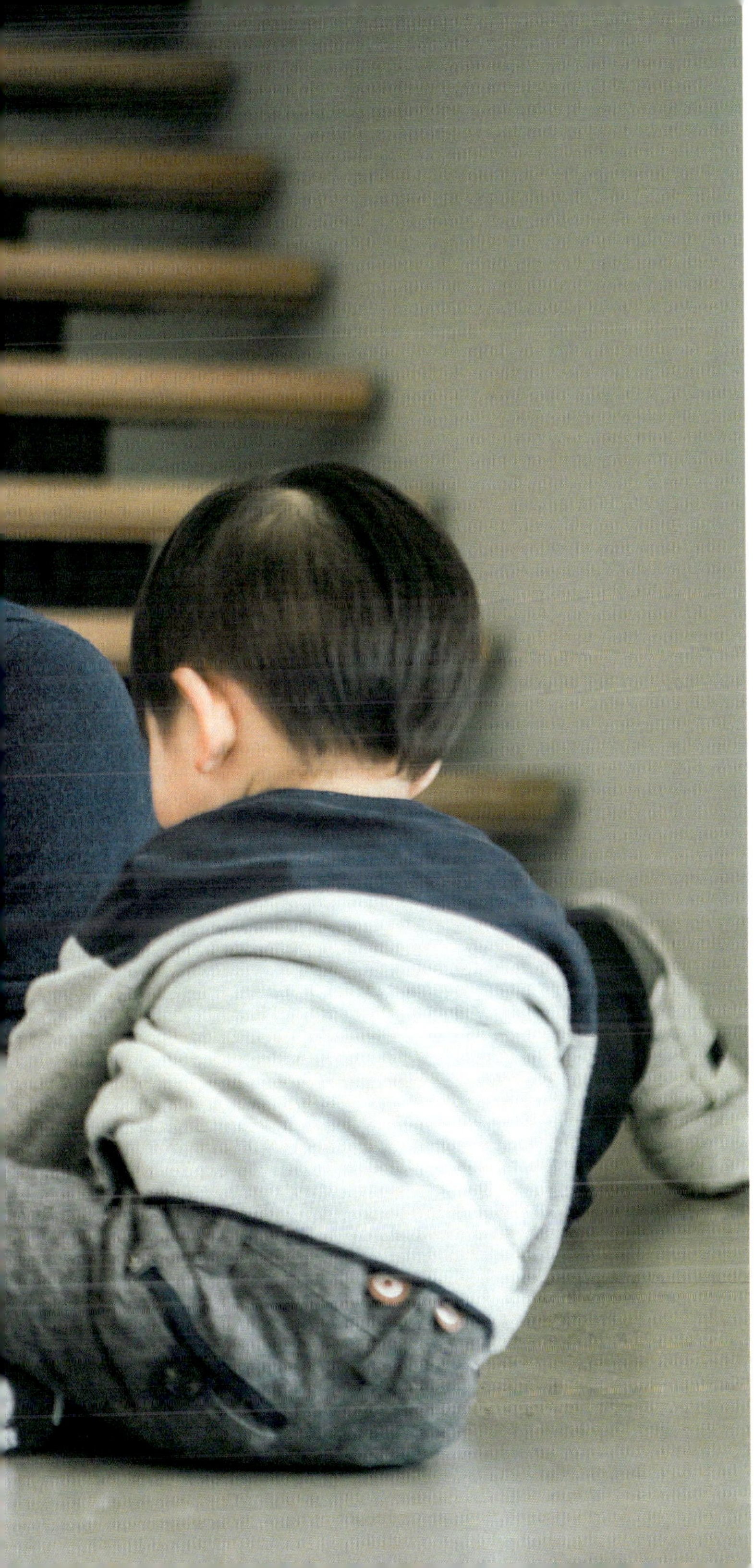

# Another parent

Encourage my dad or other parent and significant others to connect with me in their unique way, which will naturally be different to yours.

Talking, singing, cuddling, eye contact, playing and helping me feed (if I'm bottle-fed) are just some of the ways that can bring us so close together that they can recognise my signals too.

This also helps me adjust to the ways of others and provides you with much needed support.

And, as I grow

and develop...

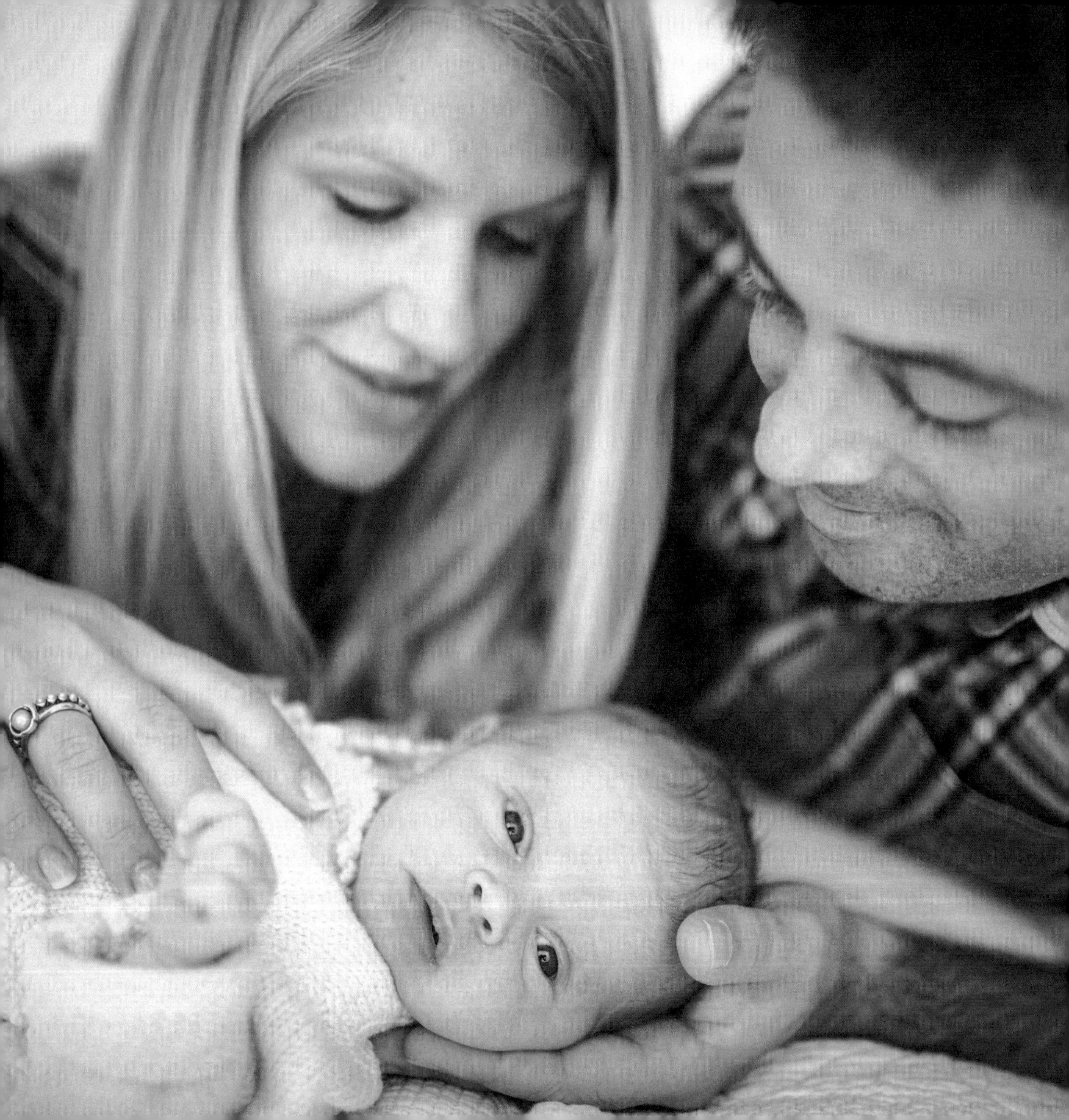

# Nourish my heart

Love, respect, kindness and forgiveness—
show me how to live these heart-nourishing ways.

The more you do this, the more they matter to me and become like my internal compass to guide me throughout my days.

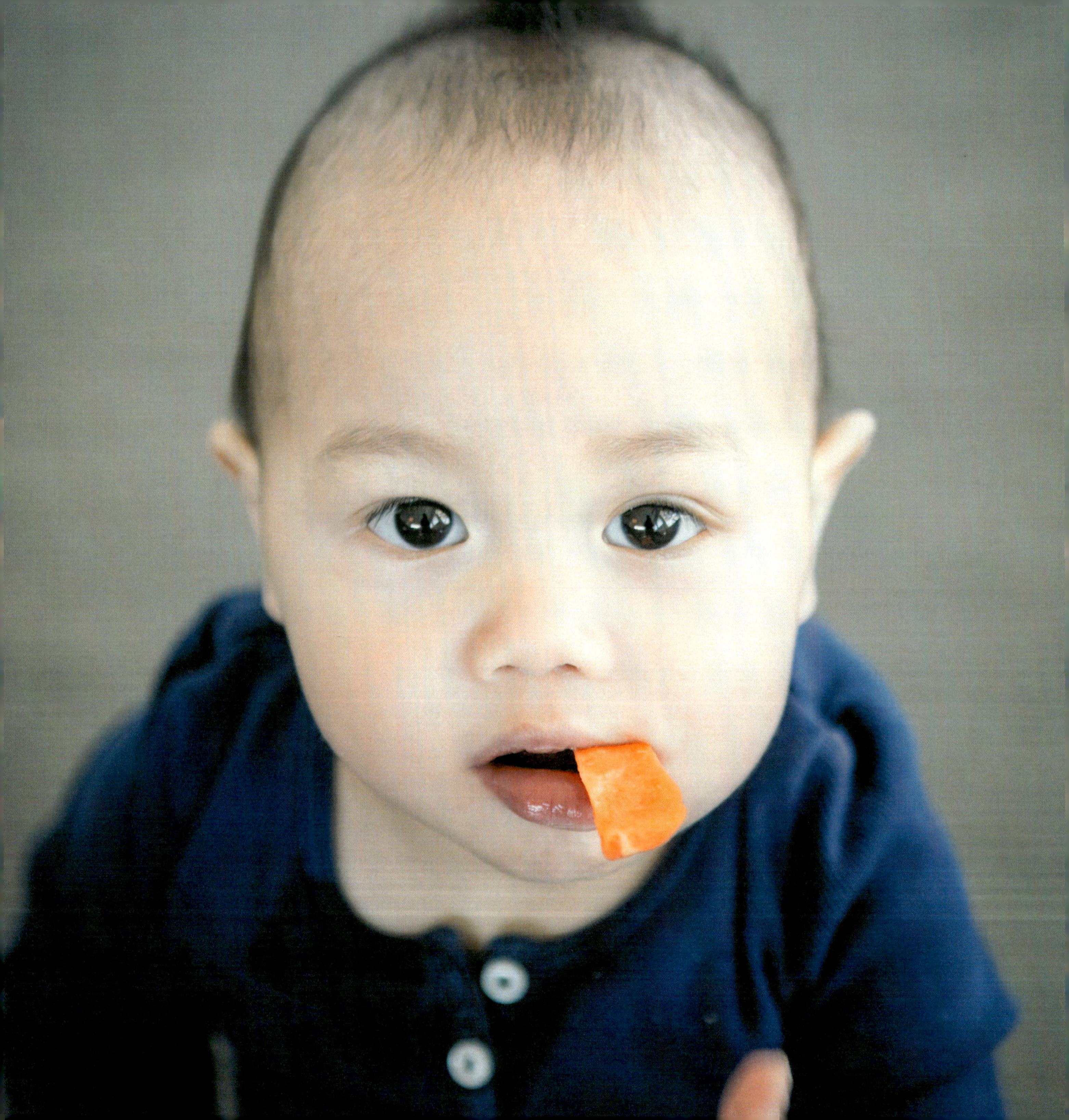

# Nourish my body

Feed me food and drinks that are fresh and wholesome.

What I eat affects how I grow and how I act.

Best of all, your healthy choices are most likely to become mine for years to come.

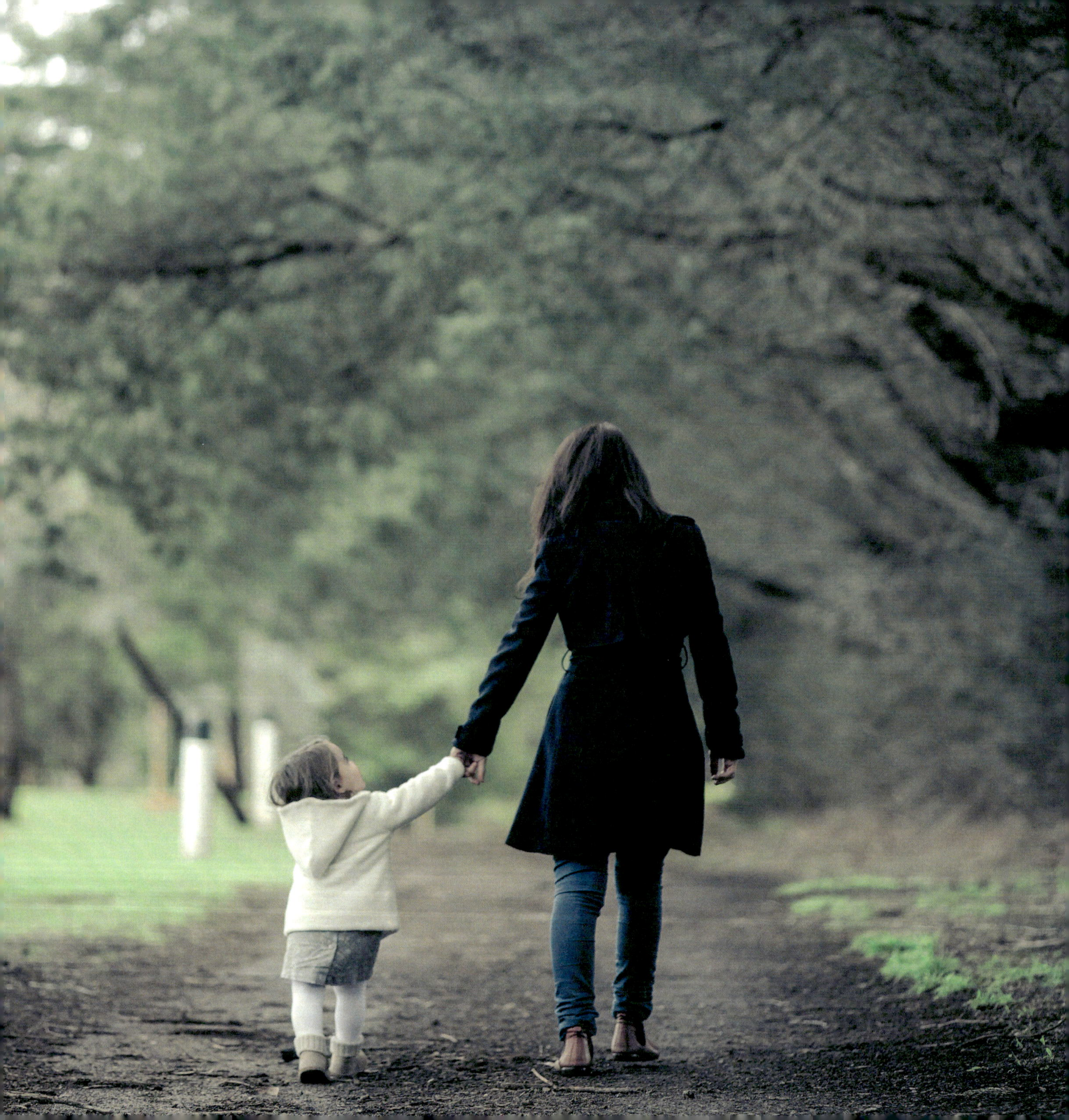

# Mother Nature helps and heals

Keep me in touch with Mother Nature—
to breathe in fresh air, feel grass tickling my toes,
and see clouds in the sky when I look up high.

Let me explore in her space what my body can do and help my eyesight develop the ability to see near and far.

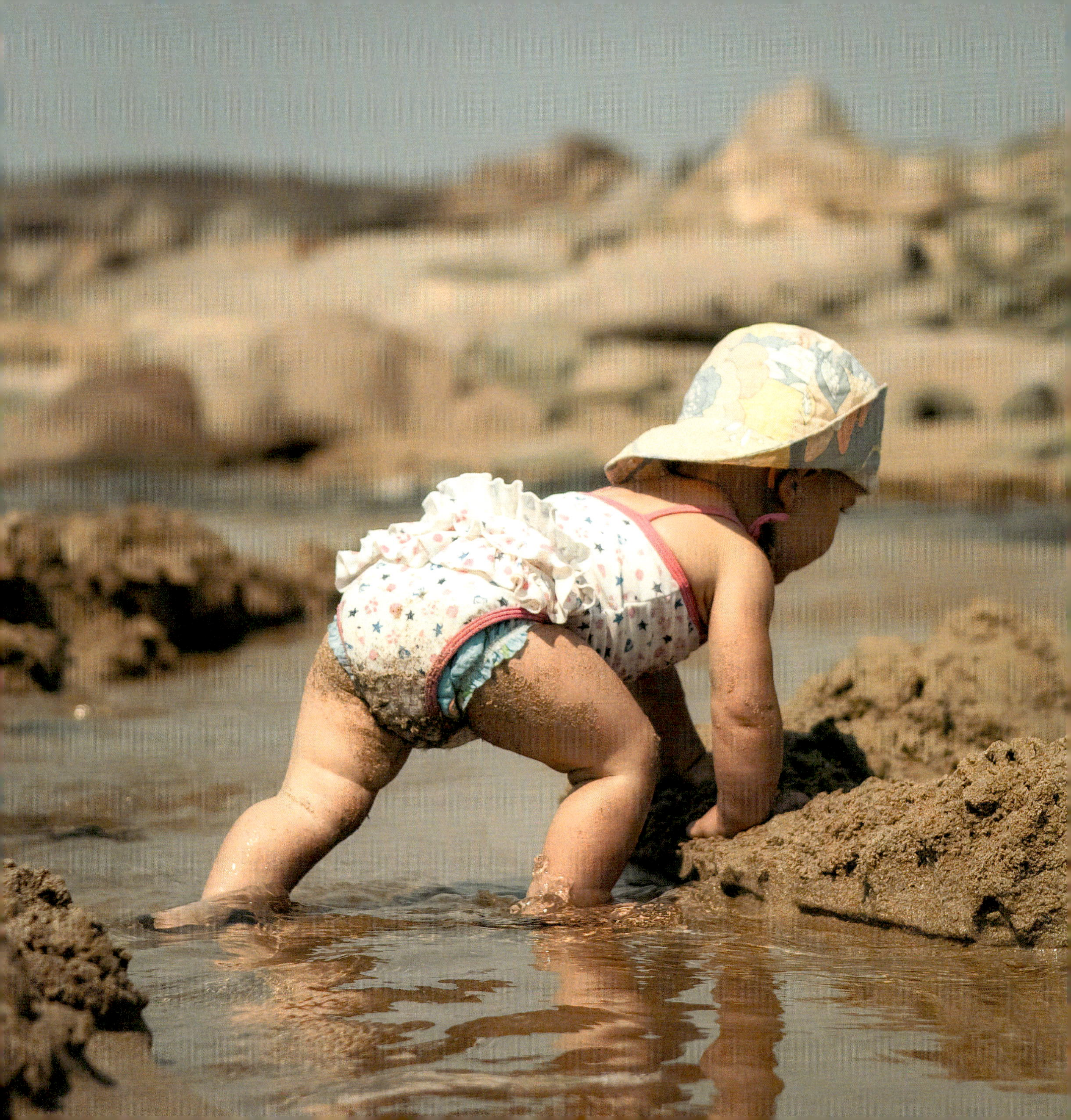

# Heading out and back

I'm busting to venture out, too far some times.

Welcome me back to your open arms, to reset until I'm ready to explore again.

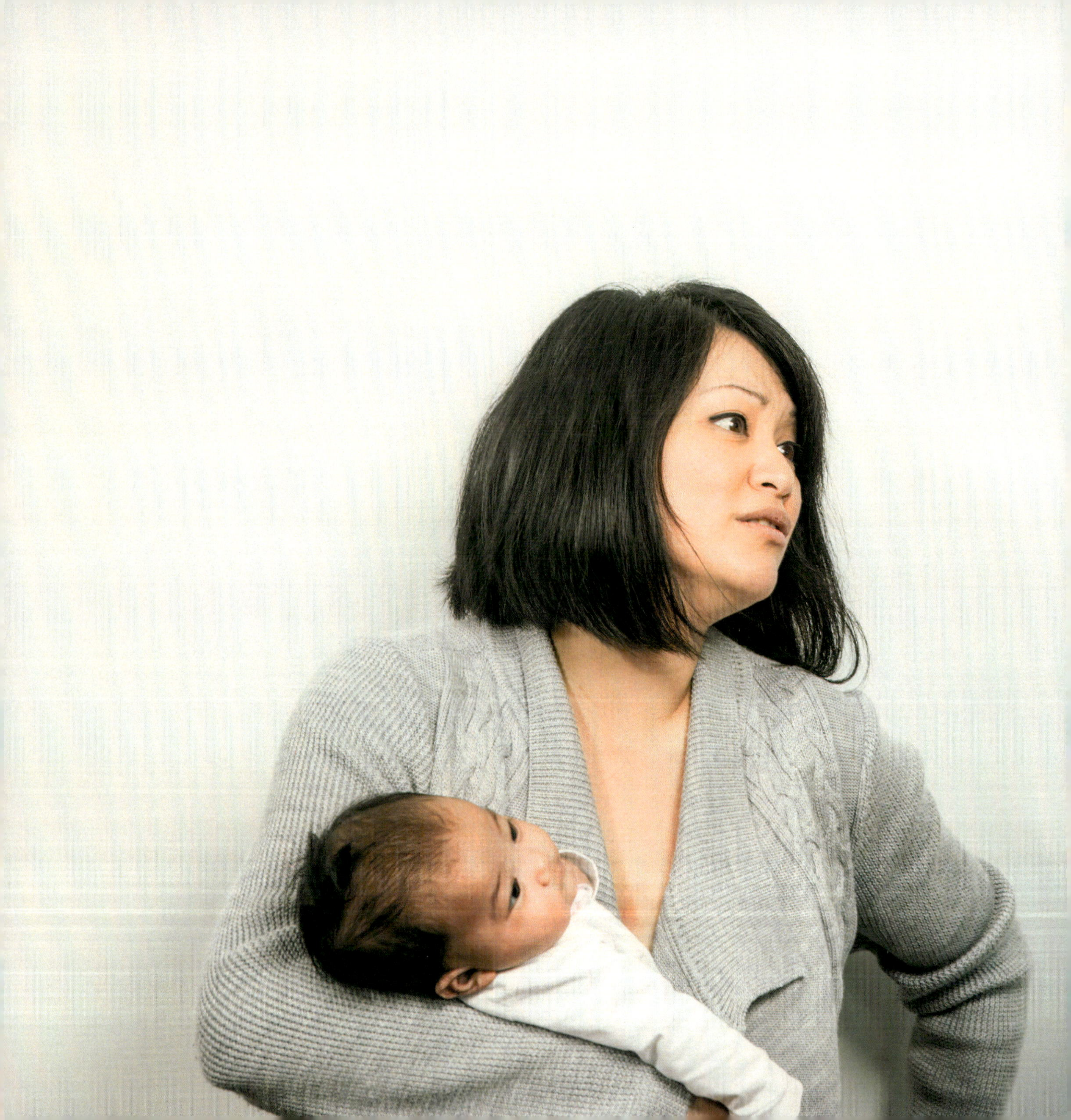

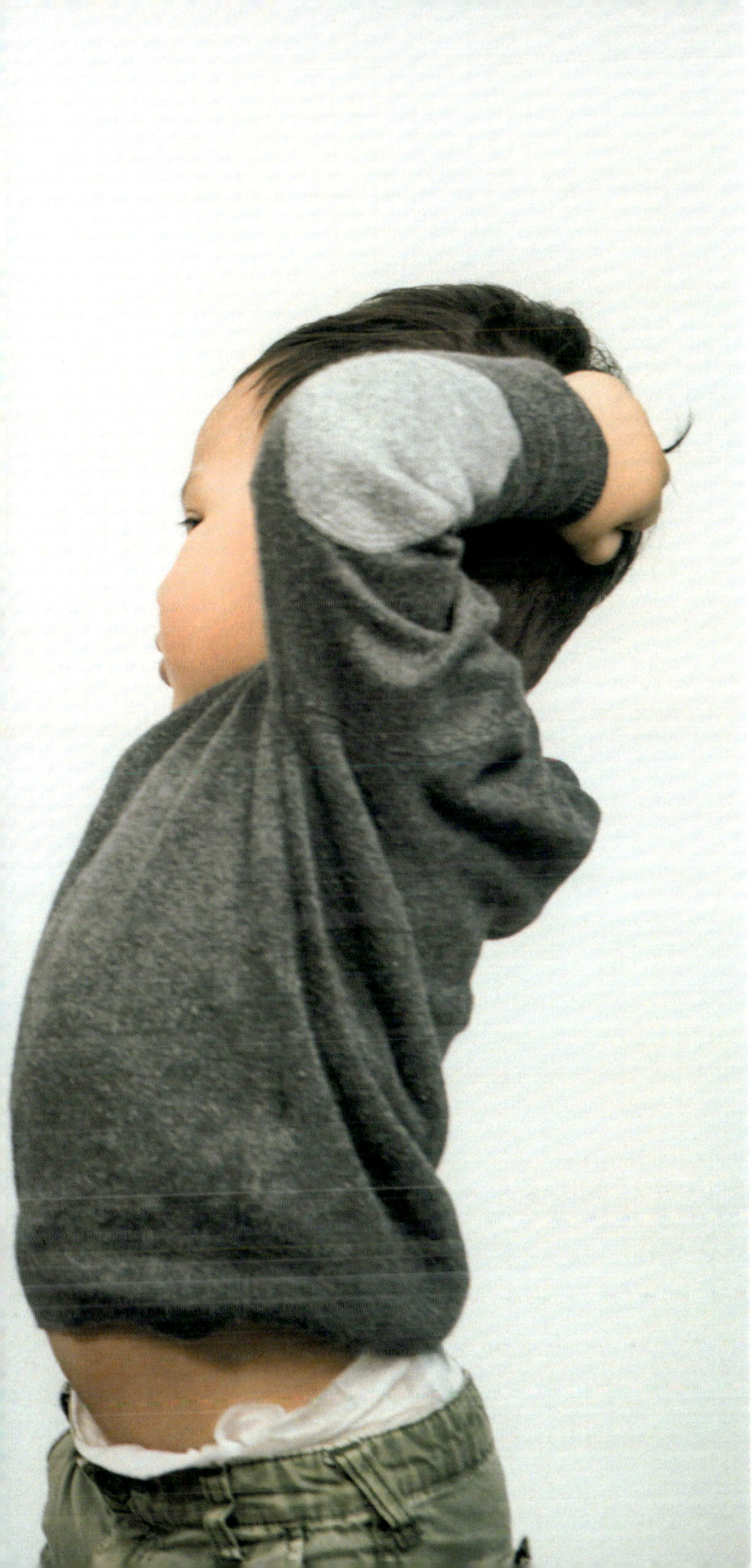

# 'No' is okay

Because you are the adult, and I'm the child, you need to make the important and sometimes tough decisions.

It is okay to say "No" to me calmly.

Show me how to do things that are good for others and me.

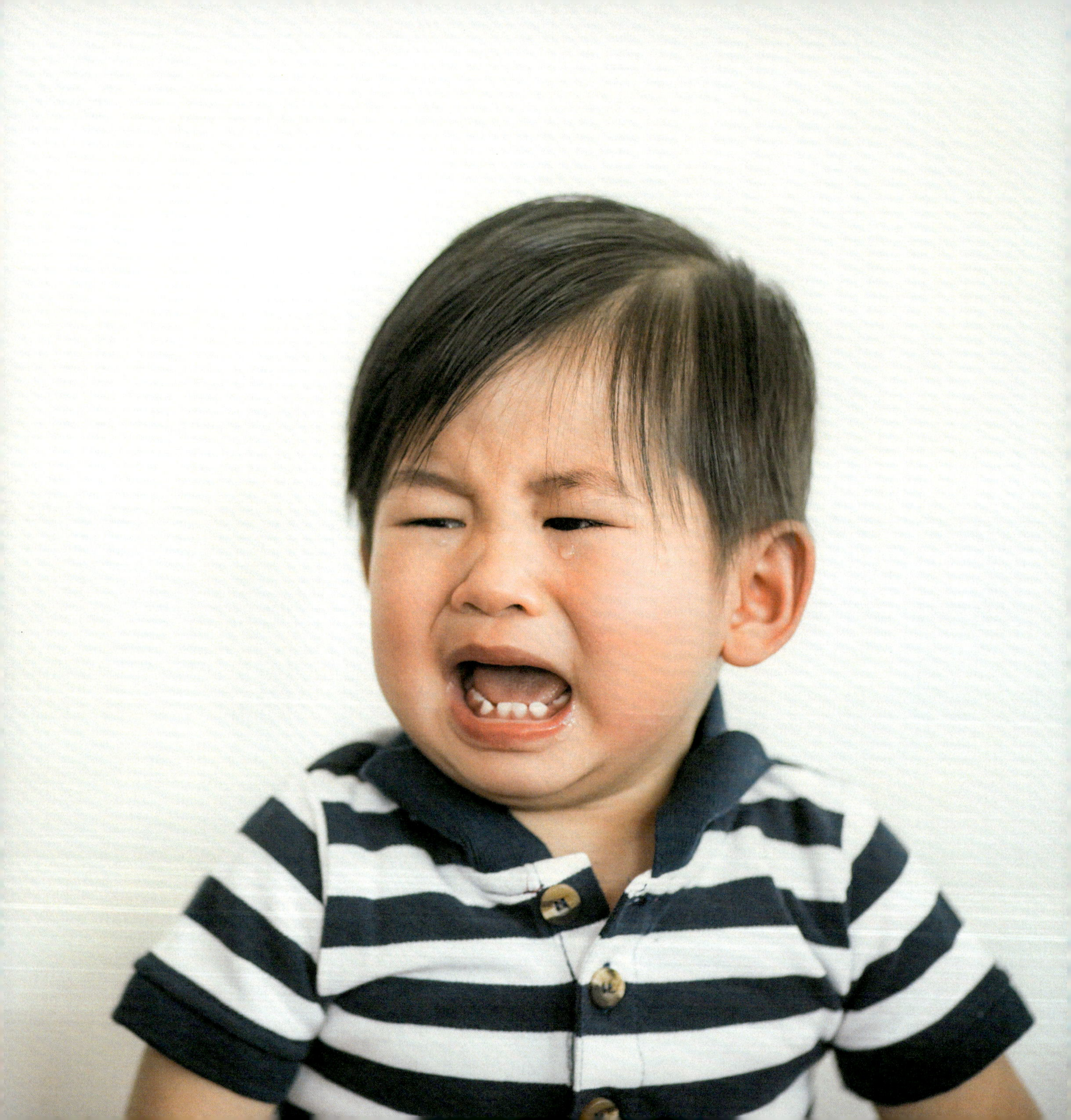

# Big feelings

Help me ride the waves of big emotions like anger and over-excitement, validating what I feel.

Overwhelming feelings can leave me horribly uncomfortable inside. I might even throw a tantrum because it's my way of trying to get them out when I don't know what else to do.

I really need you to stay by my side calmly and patiently wait until I settle.

By showing me you aren't afraid of my big feelings, I won't be either. I'll settle more quickly.

A hug when I'm ready lets me know even though I was distressed I am always lovable.

Once I'm calm, help me work through what was bothering me. All this helps me begin to manage my emotions a critical skill that you can teach me and model yourself.

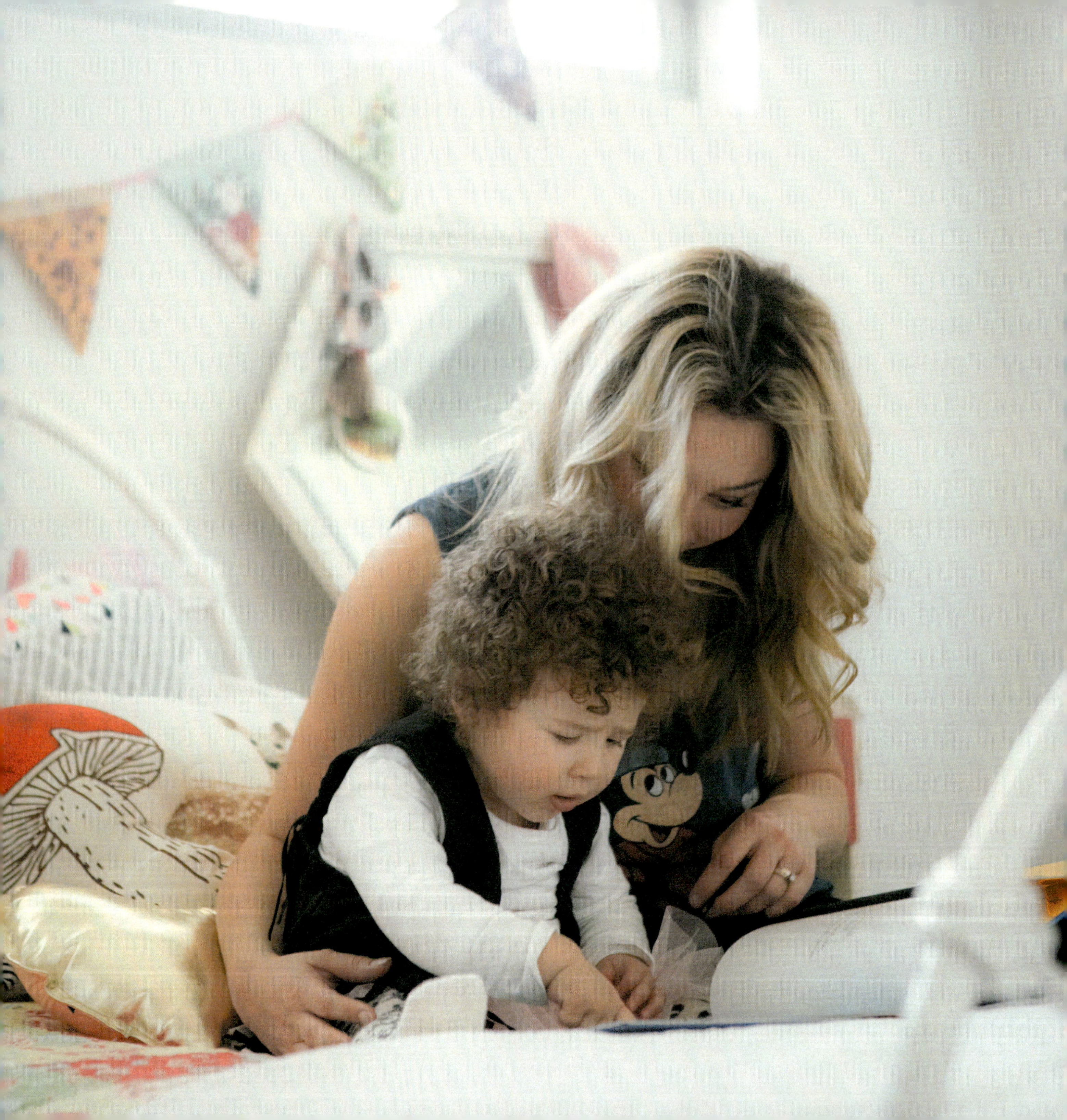

# Preparing my way

Your encouragement and praise of my efforts makes me feel like I can fly and builds my self-confidence, one of the greatest gifts you can give to me.

Be my coach rather than critic.

Believe in me when I find it hard to believe in myself.

Help me reignite my light within should it dim.

Give me just enough assistance to keep me progressing ahead.

If this becomes your way, as I find myself in more challenging times, I'll keep my ears open to what you have to say.

It may not always seem like I'm listening but I will hear and take in what I can and need at the time, to get me going again.

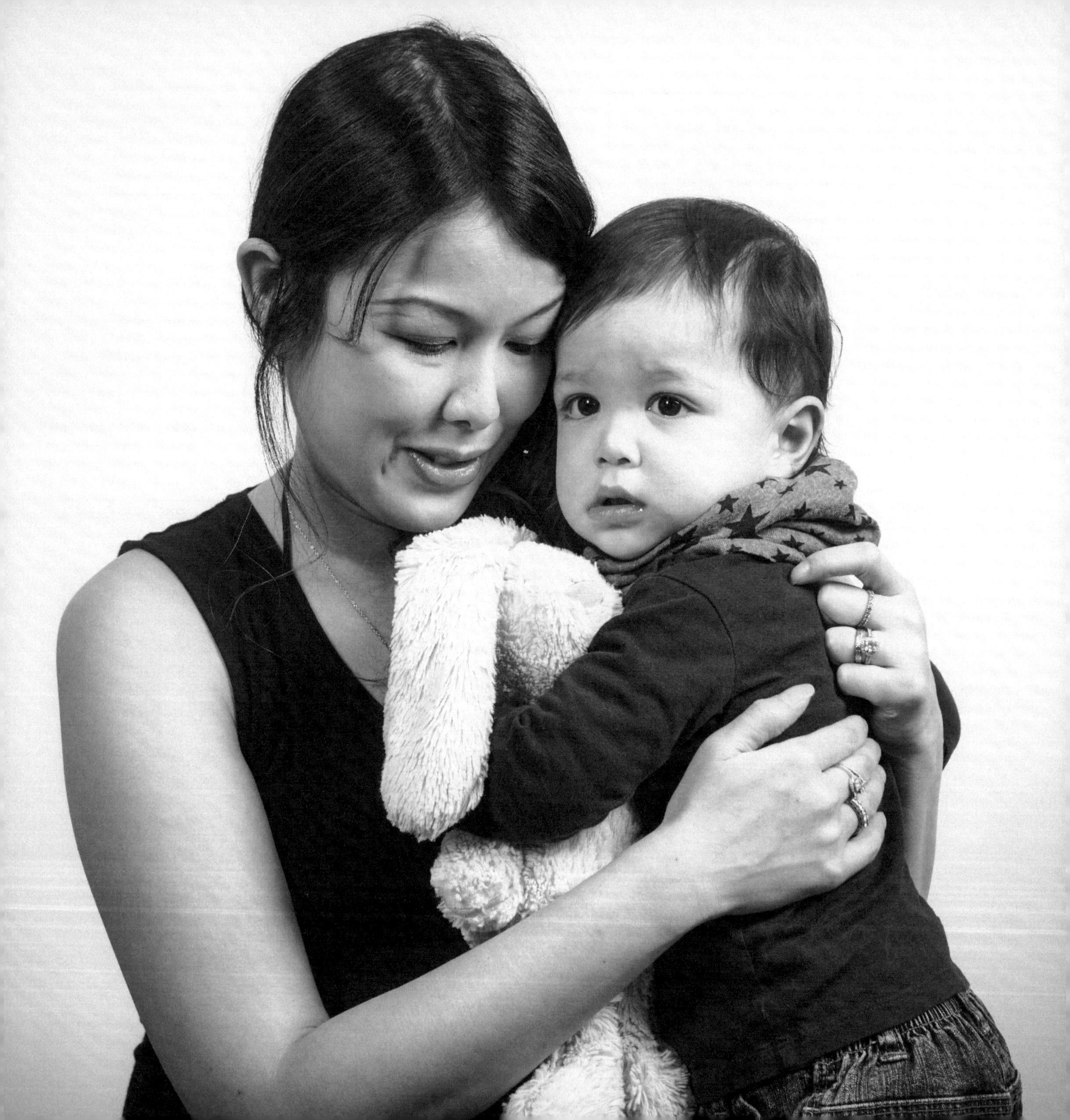

# Welcome my mistakes

Mistakes mean I've tried and like you, I'm not perfect. Your acknowledgement of my effort will more likely encourage me to try again.

Sometimes I will achieve a lot and other times not... and that's okay.

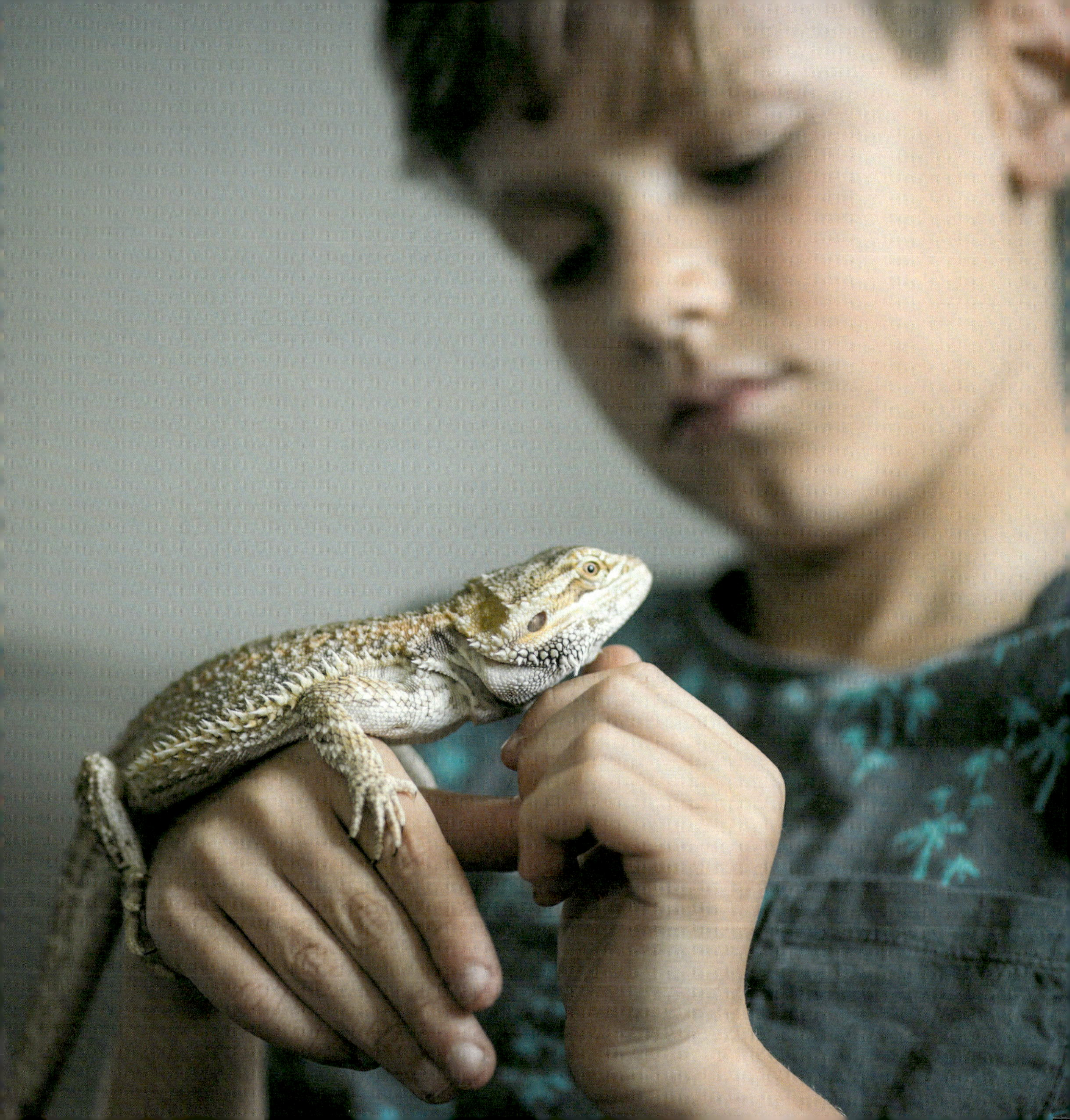

# I am whom I am

Be curious about and show interest in what I choose to do, especially when it's different to what you do. That way my individuality can shine without shame.

After all, there is no one ME-er than me.

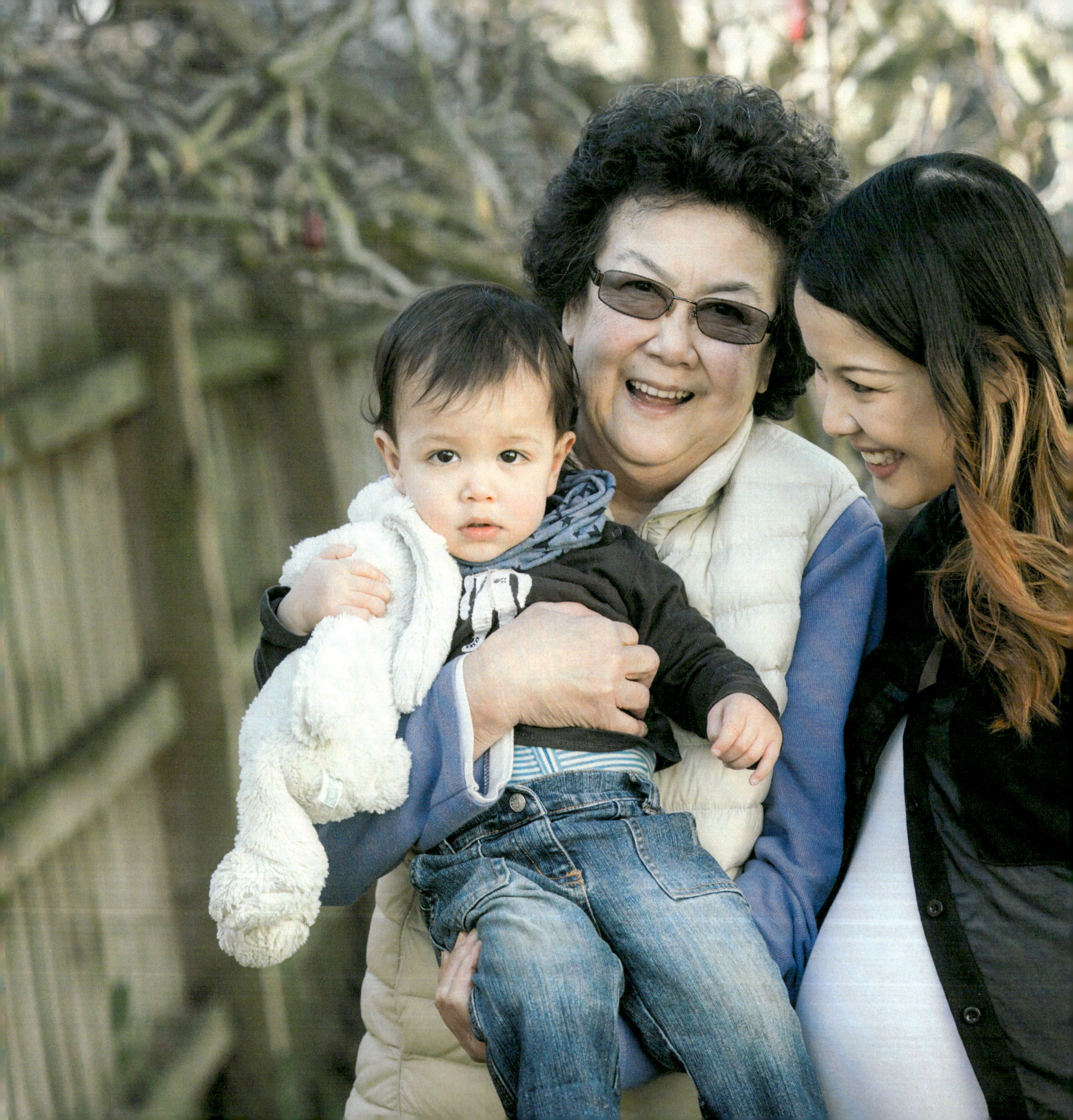

# It takes a village to raise a child

Build around me a group of caring and nurturing people, to support you, watch over me and to enrich my world.

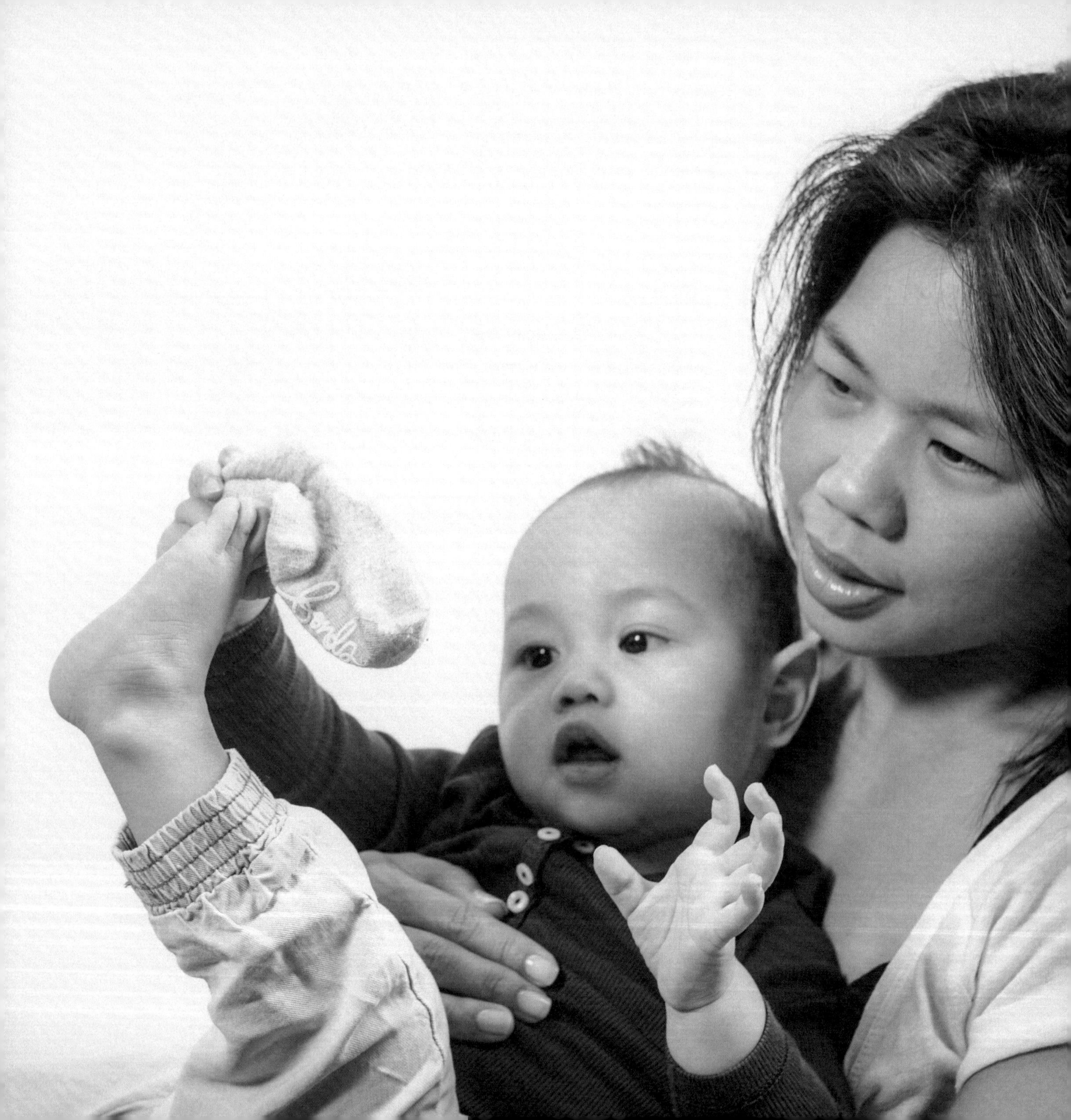

# Don't do for me what I can do for myself

I want to have a go. Let me try things my way, to test my abilities and build resilience in trying again after not getting it right the first time.

It might not be perfect or the way you'd do things.

Acknowledge my effort more than the outcome to boost my self-confidence and willingness to try more complex things.

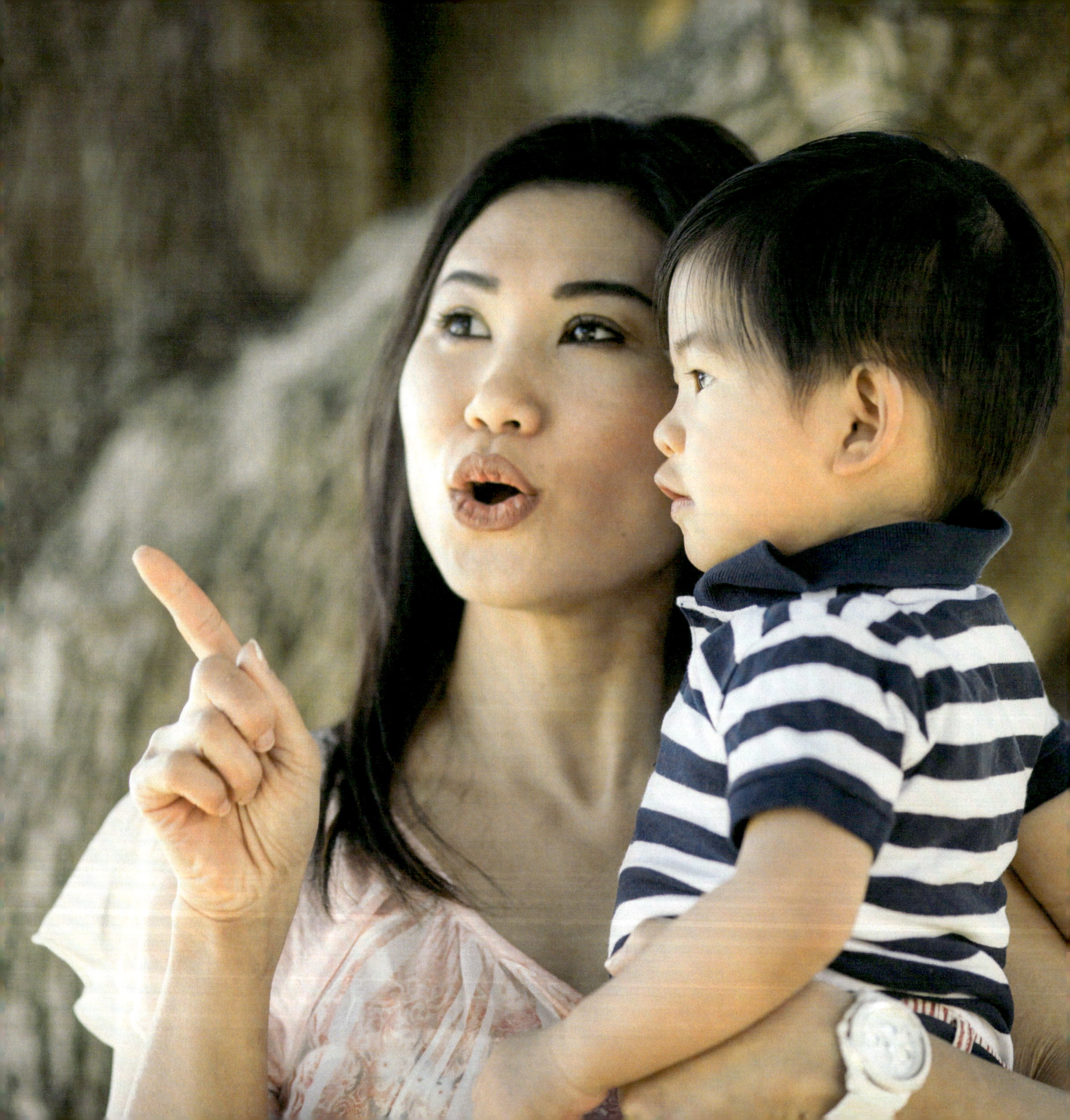

# Misbehaviour? Ask, don't tell

I am yet to develop understanding of rules and boundaries so it's inevitable that I'll break or cross them unintentionally. If my behaviour is causing problems, guide me to change my ways in an environment of safety and security rather than threats and punishment that only serve to build anger and resentment in the long run.

Stay calm and have curiosity about what I am doing. Be like a detective to work out what could be going on for me. Withhold judgment and connect with me by *saying what you see*. For example, "You two seem to want to play with the same toy."

Involve me in problem solving by *setting the limits*. "Only one person can play with the toy at a time." *Provide limited choices* that you'd be happy to live with. "Would you like to pick another toy or choose a storybook for me to read to you until it's your turn?" Questions that lead me to make wise decisions empower me.

When I change my behaviour for the better, acknowledge what I can do. For example, "Thank you for sharing your toys. You both look happy now."

If I can't help myself and neither can you, seek outside guidance so things don't escalate unnecessarily.

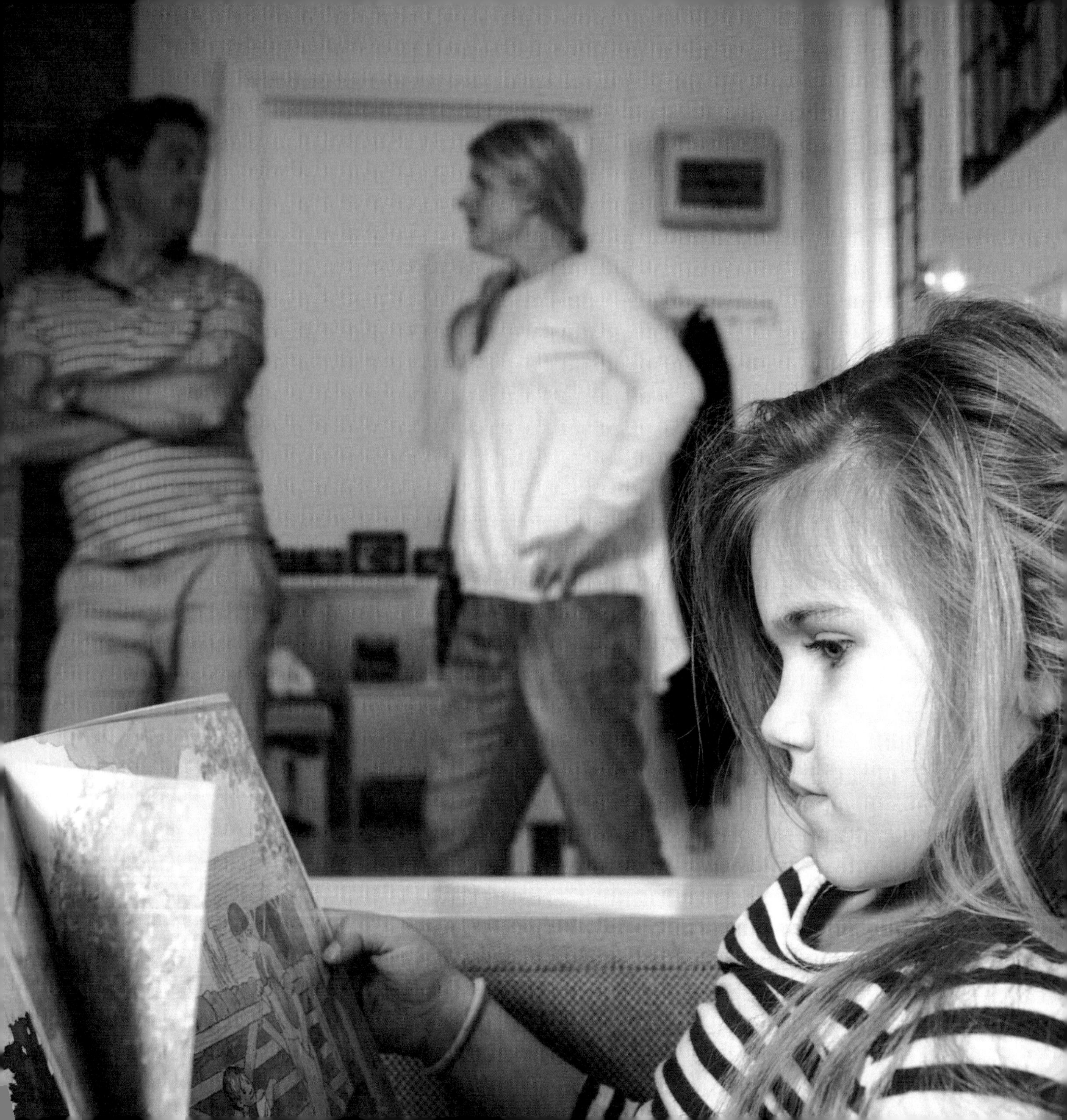

# Relating to others

The way you interact with your intimate one in front of me, has a greater effect on my being than how you treat me.

This is also likely to become my template for my future adult relationships.

It's okay to respectfully disagree with others in front of me, just remember to demonstrate how you work through heated moments to restore harmony.

Keep adult business to yourselves because I only have a child's brain and need it to be free from adult worries to enjoy the childhood I deserve.

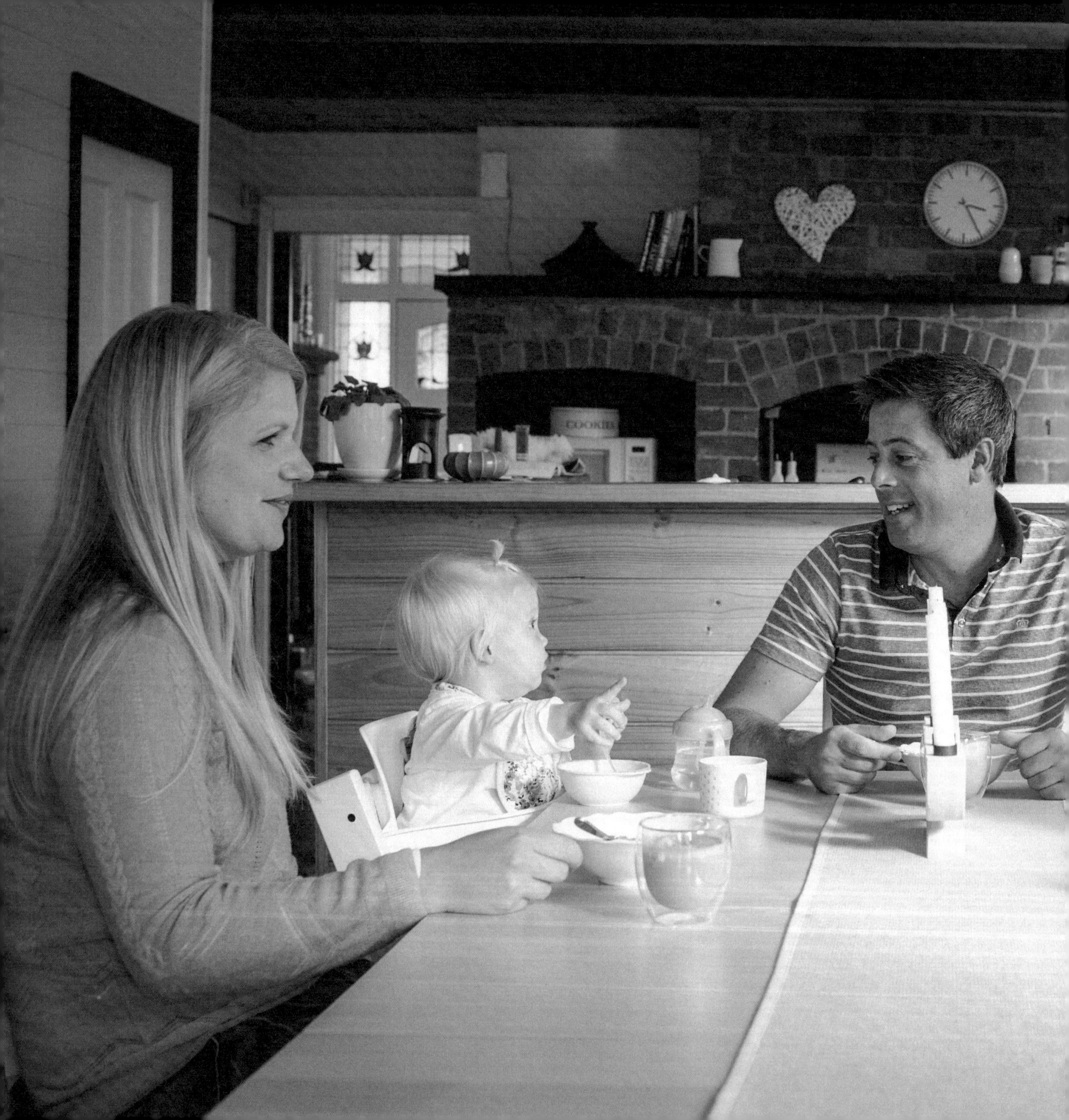

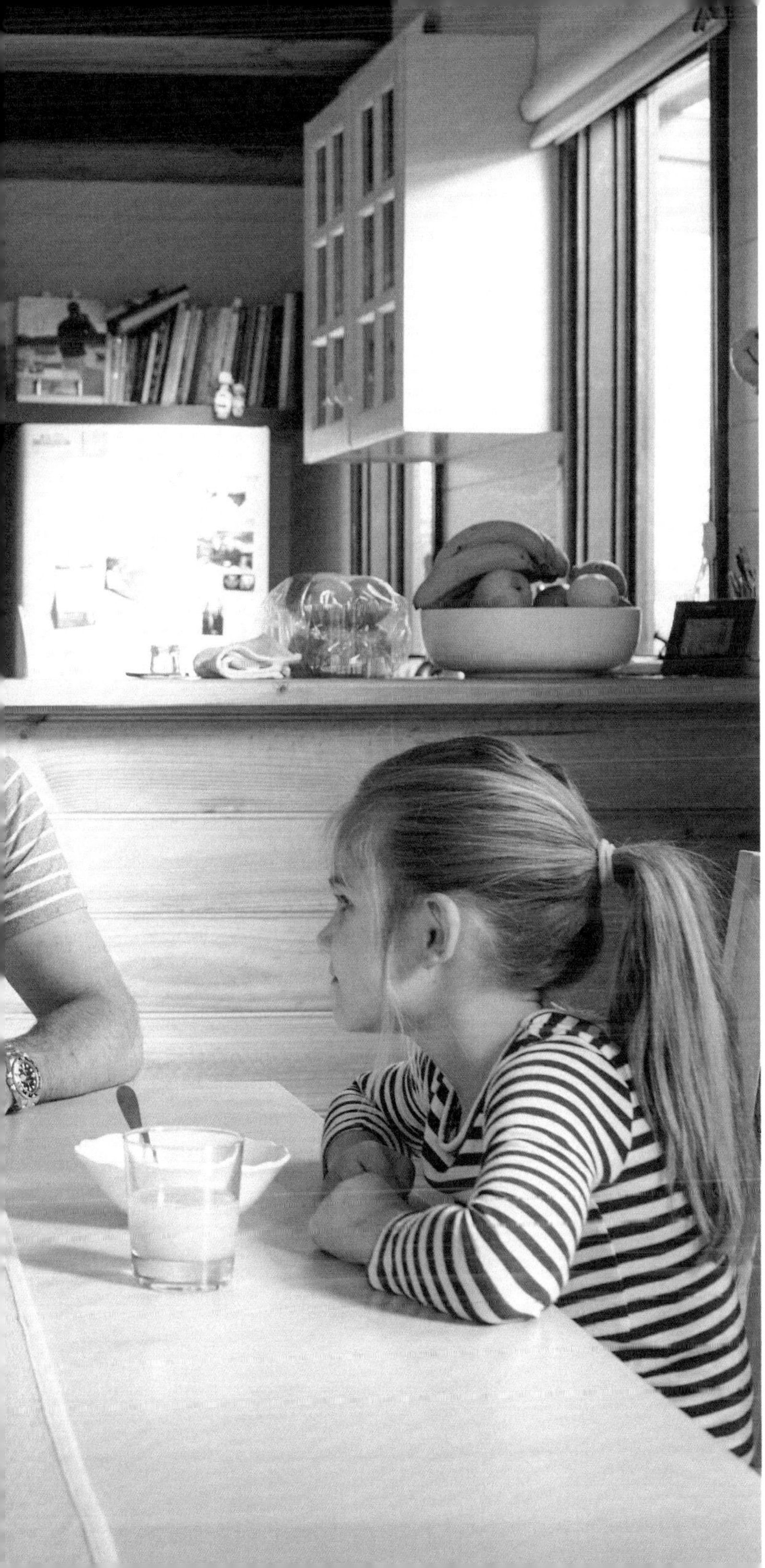

# Come to the table

From cradle to grave,
sharing of meals
nourishes my body,
heart and mind.

In our busy world,
this one regular time
slows us down:
to connect, listen, chat
about our day and
be grateful for each
other and everything
in our lives.

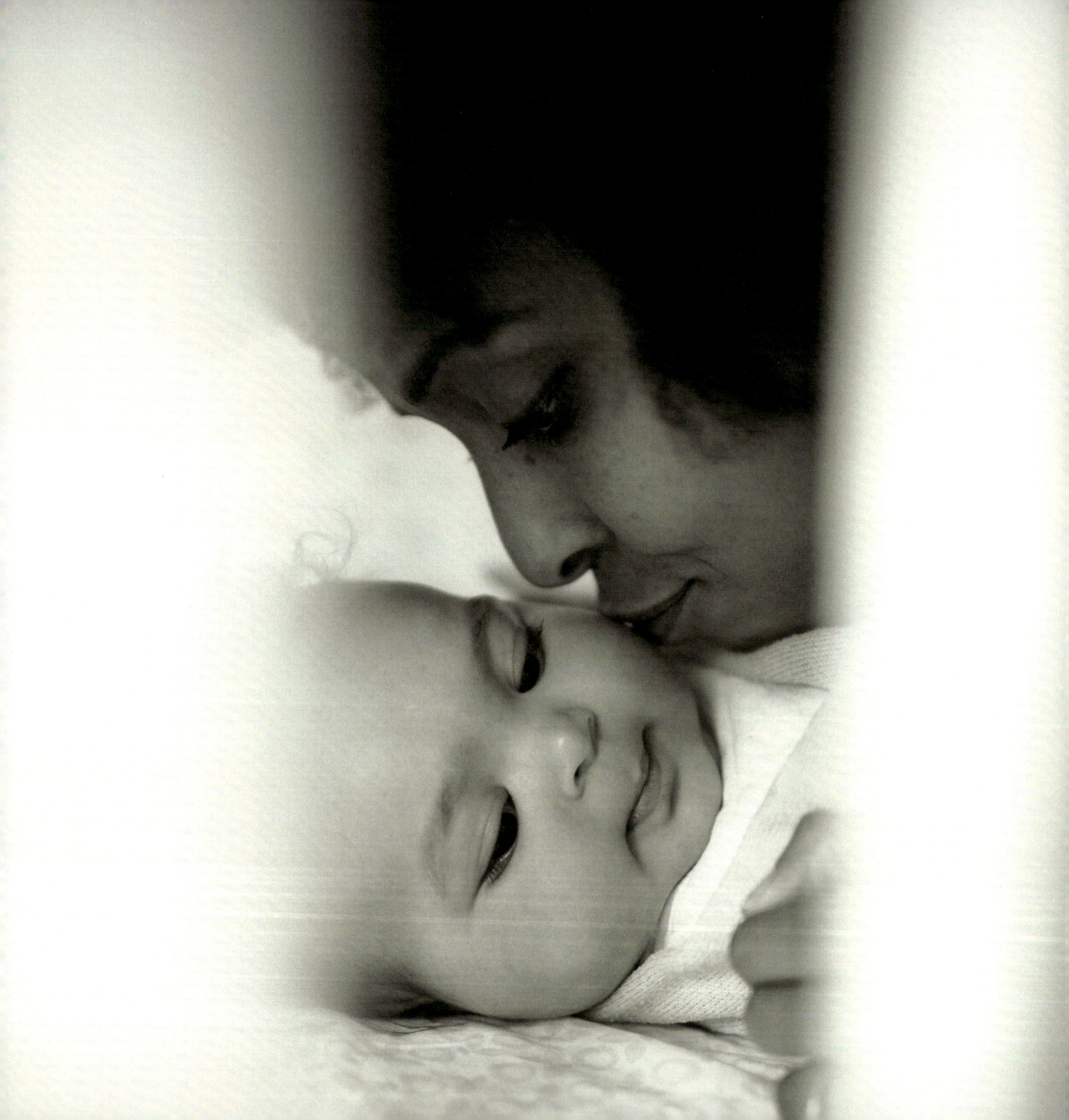

# A Kiss goodnight and some sparkle for the morrow

When I lay my head upon my pillow to rest, let's take a few minutes for just you and me.

Maybe read to me or when I'm a little older have a wee chat about what was important to me that day, to find out what I'm grateful for and what I hope for tomorrow.

Add a little sparkle with your kiss or a cuddle, a special song or a face stroke and of course, an "I love you."

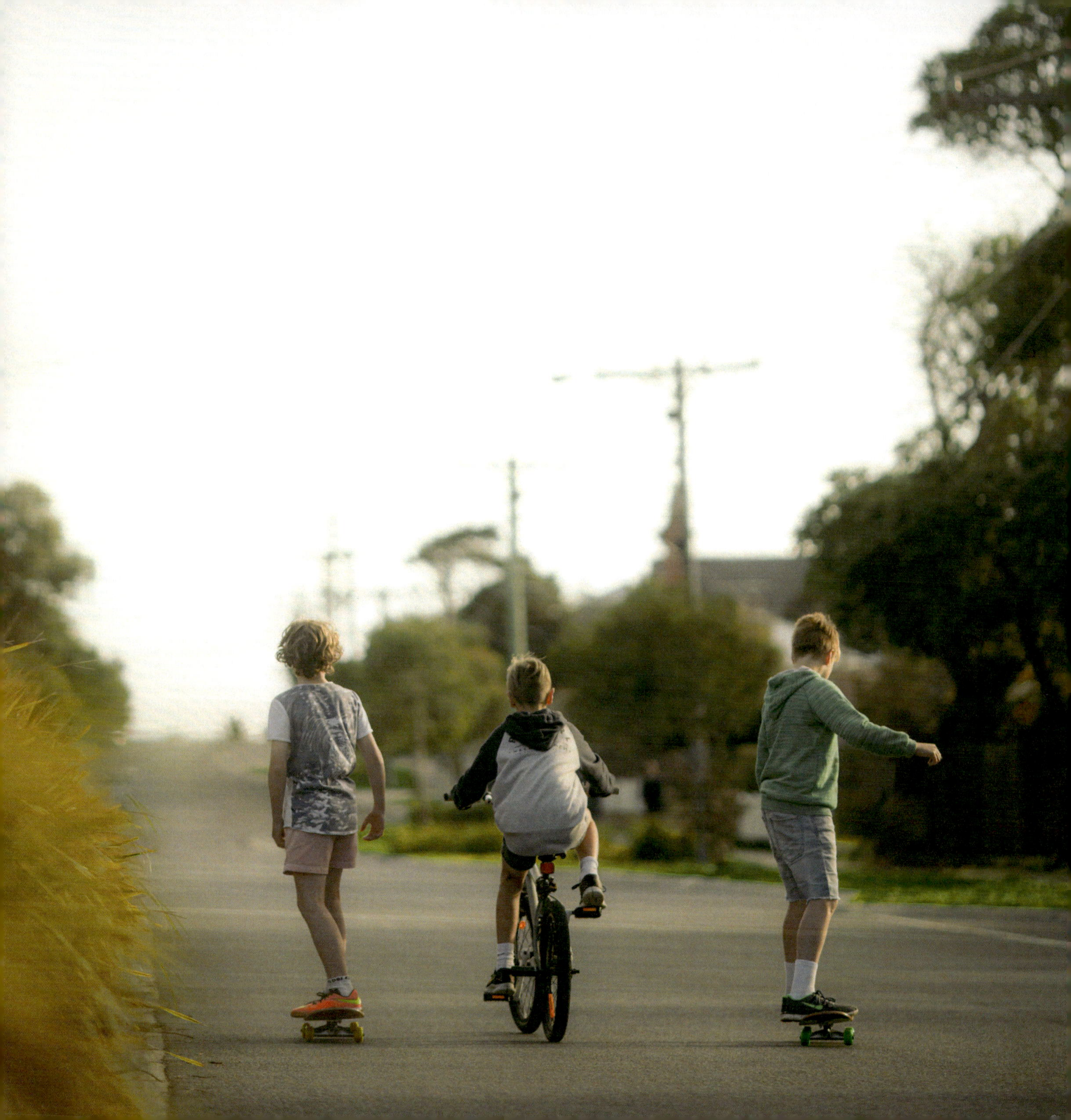

# In search of self

As I move through adolescence, I'll shift my focus away from you to others, in search of who I am.

It will be your love that I hold in my heart that keeps me most on track.

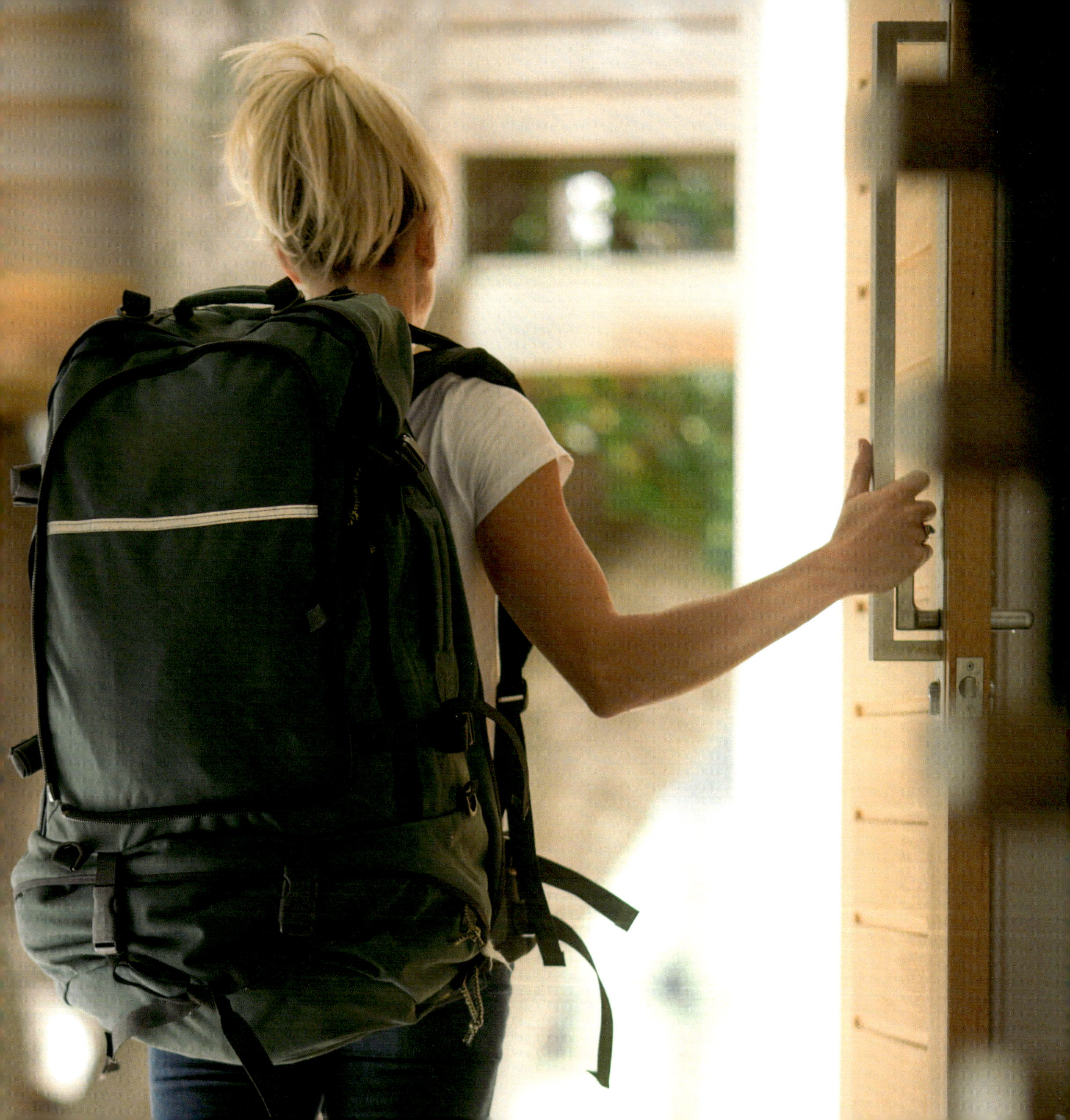

# Just for a while then off I go

Our close days will seem to fly by... then I'm off in the world to take my place...

I hope with your blessings powering the wings of my dreams.

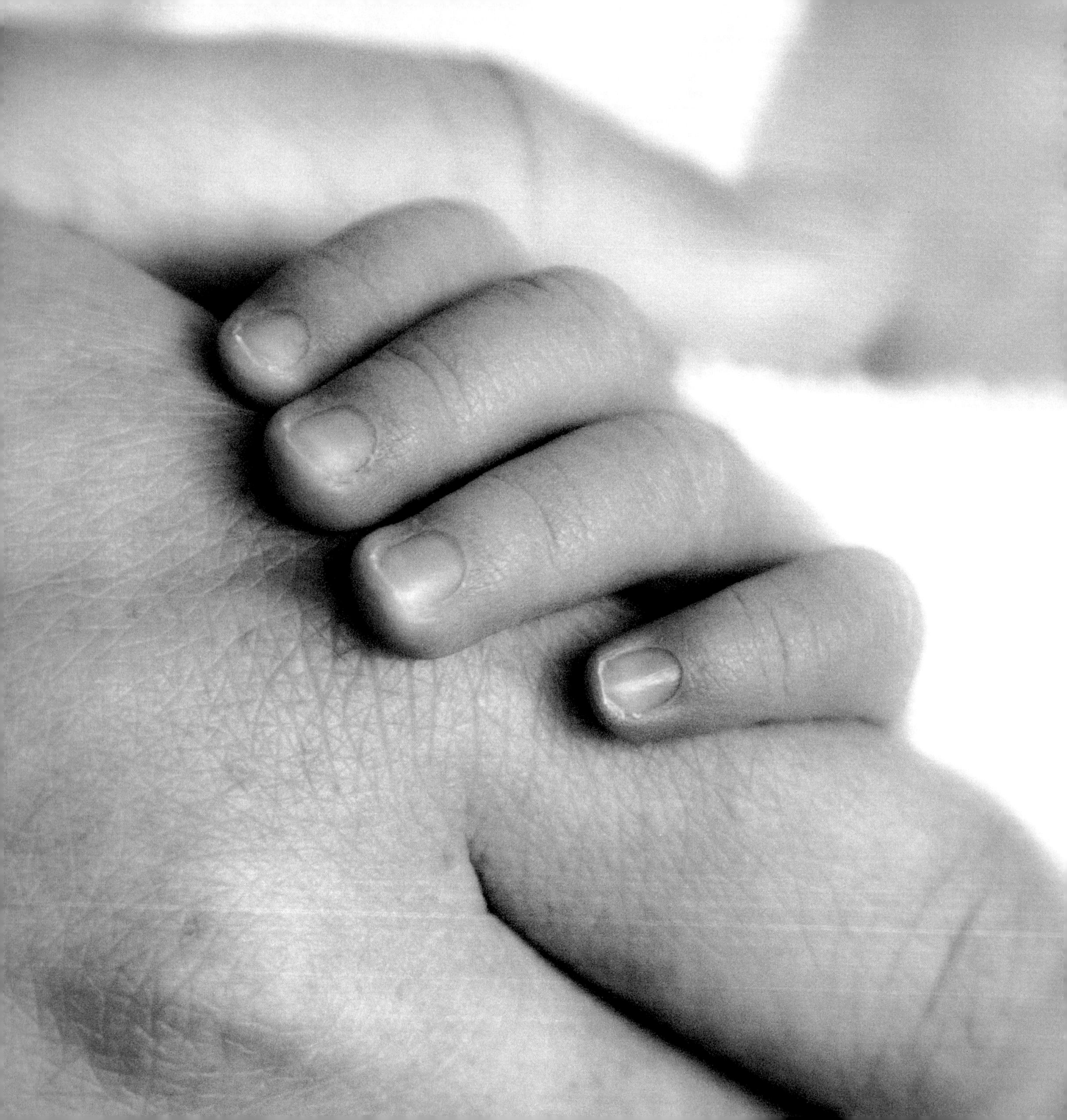

# In years to come

And if it comes time for me to have my own children, I'll know that...

Through my eyes, baby sees me, just as I did you.

And our hearts will connect... forever.

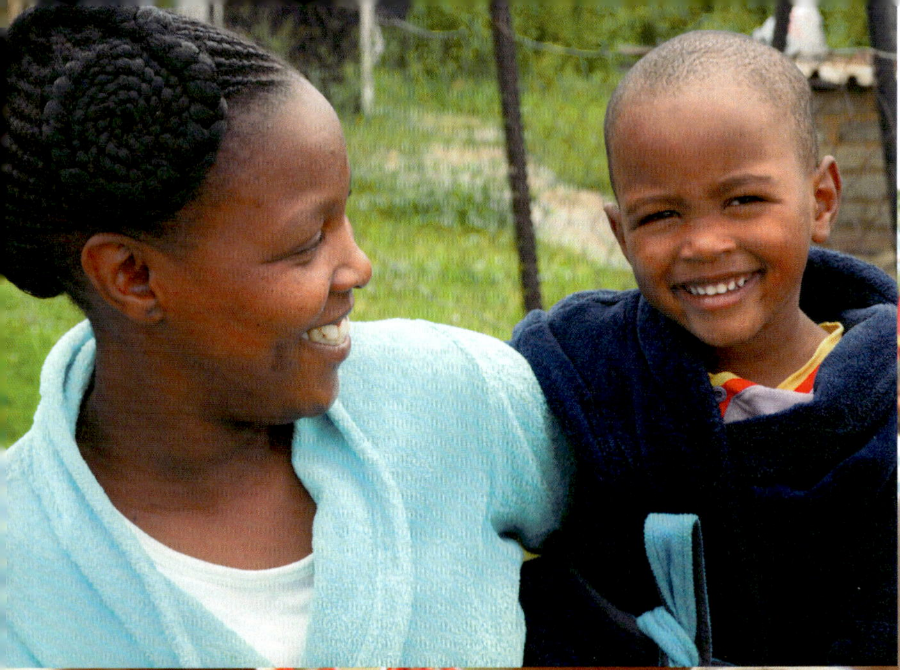

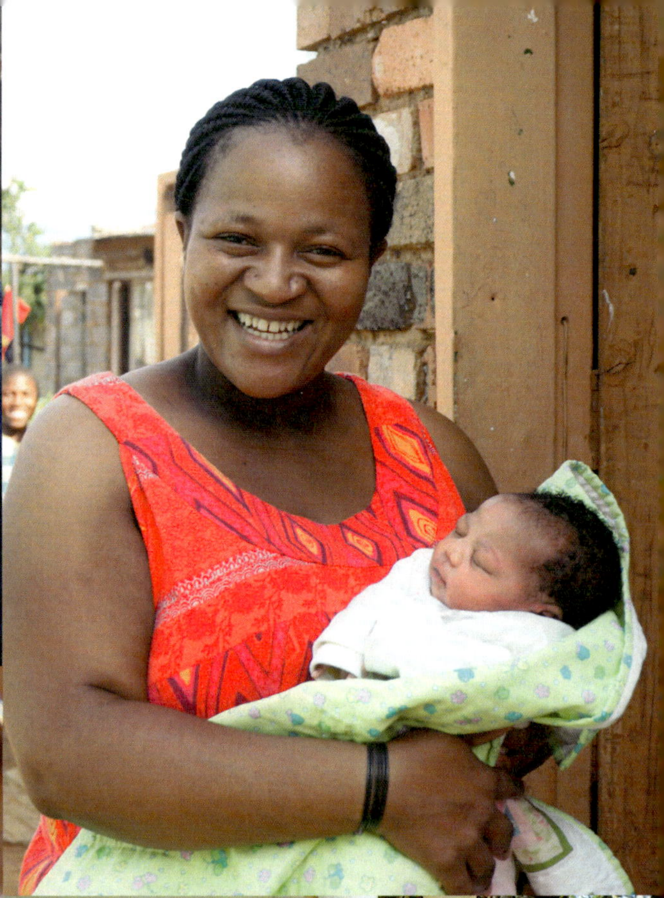

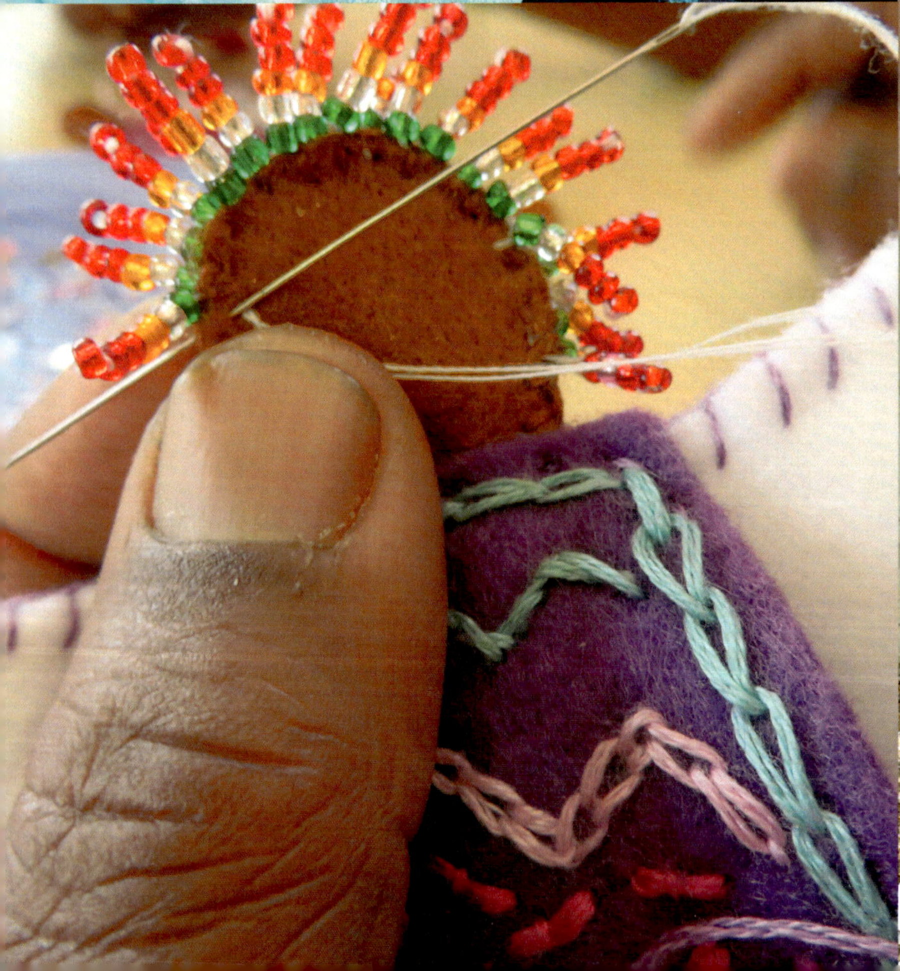

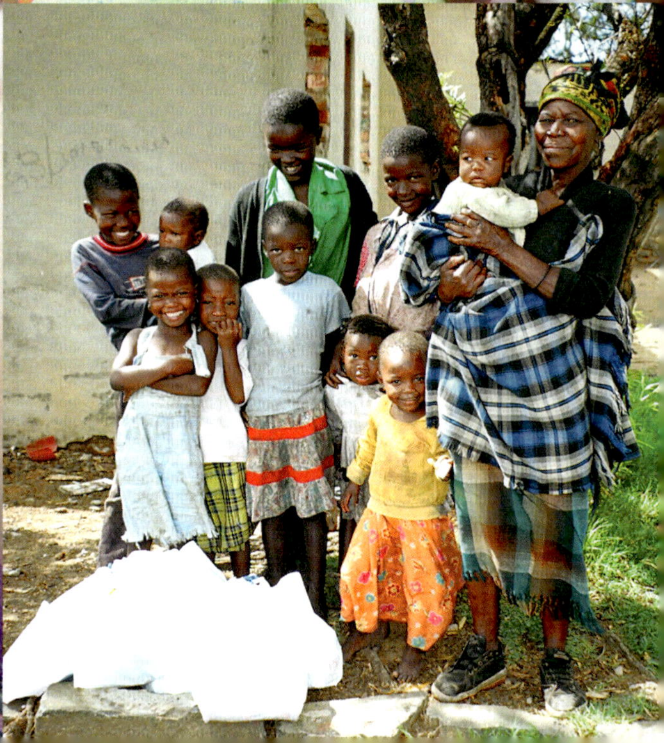

# The Kopanang Project, South Africa

"Kopanang is a place where hearts find accepting and nurturing love in a community that stands by one another through chaos, loss of every conceivable kind, poverty, and conversely, a place where all are one and support one another to be the best they can be. They celebrate life even in their struggles with enormous courage and faith, and sing like angels!"

—Sister Sheila Flynn (Founder, Director).

Visit ***Kopanang.org*** for more information, to buy their products or to donate.

CPSIA information can be obtained
at www.ICGtesting.com
Printed in the USA
BVXC01n1258231216
5028BVAU00002B/4
* 9 7 8 1 9 2 5 5 1 6 3 2 6 *